TABLE O⟩

M000222424

ABOUT THE AUTHOR

Dr. Tom Owen is a licensed professional counselor and certified fitness trainer. He has been helping people get in shape for over 30 years. Dr. Owen won his first power lifting championship weighing 165 pounds in 1970. He gained 130 pounds of muscle over the next 15 years to become a 300-pound super heavyweight champion, setting numerous world records. He is pictured in the *1987 Guinness Book of World Records* as a professional strongman.

Over a period of three decades, Tom has won dozens of titles in both power lifting and bodybuilding. In 1988, he won the Master Mr. Alabama Bodybuilding Championship at a weight of 245 pounds, and he has continued to sculpt his body into a lean, national master's physique champion, briefly going under 3% body fat for competition! He is the current Great South Power Lifting Champion, and a first runner-up in both the Master Mr. U.S.A. and Mr. America.

While taking his weight down to 228 pounds for competition, Tom personally knows the importance of eating lean and staying lean. This book explains how these simple principles can work for you.

Tom has five degrees, including a B.S. in Health and an Ed.S. in Counseling Psychology from the University of Alabama at Birmingham. He also has a Doctorate in Christian Counseling.

Tom is featured regularly on national television, most recently the *Jay Leno Show* on NBC and *The Crook & Chase Show* on CBS. He has also been featured on the Fox Network as "Mr. Muscle," as well as on other national news and talk shows. Tom has his own TV and radio program entitled, "American Fitness" and "Tom's Tips for Health." These were syndicated throughout the Southeast for several years.

Currently, he is the owner of American Fitness Gym in Birmingham, Alabama.

Since 1975, Tom has been dedicated to helping hurting or homeless youth, and he is currently the Founder and Director of the Alabama Youth Home—a place where youngsters with problems can live and learn to grow up to be healthy and wholesome adults.

The Alabama Youth Home benefits from the proceeds of this book.

CONTRIBUTING AUTHOR

David Berman has a Master's Degree in Physical Therapy and is a Licensed Physical Therapist practicing in Birmingham, Alabama. He is currently working toward an Advanced Master's Degree in Orthopedic Manual Therapy (MOMT) and a Doctorate in Physical Therapy (DPT).

ACKNOWLEGEMENT

My appreciation to DonDee Crowson and Cindy Lewis for hours of typing, reading, editing, and re-editing. Their encouragement and contribution made this book possible.

DEDICATION

This book is dedicated to the boys and girls and staff at the Alabama Youth Home; to my family; to my staff and clients at American Fitness Center; to my brother Dr. G. Scott Owen who is a Master Marathon runner, College Professor and extremely knowledgeable in Fitness and Nutrition; and to all my friends, Physicians, Trainers and others who have given me knowledge and encouragement over the years.

INTRODUCTION

People find themselves out of shape, out of health, and overweight for different reasons. Many of these people have lost weight only to regain it. The information contained herein is designed to help you get where you want to be and stay there. As a psychological therapist, I am fully aware of the "food feeling connection" — the mental, emotional, and psychological aspects of weight loss. I am also aware of the hormonal challenges that people face. The simple fact is that regardless of why you are overweight or in poor health, you can improve! Simply put, use the principles outlined. There are explanations, reason, and logic, but most of all, practical advice to get you where you want to be and keep you there. You will be encouraged to take control of your health and challenged to live a healthy life-style, focusing on your behavior rather than pounds. You will find this book motivating, inspirational, and educational in your quest to become the healthiest, most fit person you can be.

Chapter One

Why Feed the Muscle and Starve the Fat?

When some people read the title of this book, they are going to assume that this is for professional bodybuilders or other aspiring athletes and may not feel they need to "feed the muscle and starve the fat." However, whether you are nine or ninety, this is exactly what you want to do. You want your body to get rid of the excess baggage, known as fat. It serves no good or useful function other than to weigh you down. On the other hand, muscle is what allows you to be mobile from infancy and for the rest of your life. There is a new medical science that is interested in helping you learn to live younger and longer, literally adding life to your years as well as years to your life. Fat does not contribute to this, muscle does. Not only do you want to get the fat off your body, but out of your arteries as well.

Anytime you think of losing weight, concentrate on losing fat, not muscle. At this point, you may not want to be a female bodybuilder or a Mr. America. I understand that. However, if you are a 5'8" man and weigh 200 pounds with 25% body fat, wouldn't you rather be 5'8", weigh 175 pounds and have 15% body fat? It just makes sense. You'll have better shape, look better, and feel better. As a personal trainer and a licensed psychological therapist, I can't tell you the number of women that have told me "I don't want to gain any muscle. I just want a better shape and to get rid of this fat on my stomach, hips, and thighs, etc." The best way to get rid of that fat is by gaining muscle. Don't worry about looking like the female bodybuilders that you see on television; it's not going to happen. What you can expect is to reduce your overall body fat, get rid of the jiggle when you walk, firm up, be stronger, have more energy, and maintain a much better body shape for the rest of your life.

Another reason that you want to gain muscle is the more muscle you have, the more metabolic you are. Metabolism is defined as the rate at which you burn calories at rest. Again, I'm not referring to becoming muscle bound, but developing firmness, tone, and strength, as well as a better physique through gaining muscle and getting rid of fat. That's should be your goal. It's never too late to start. I have a friend who is 84 years old. She never touched a weight until she was 79, and she recently bench pressed 90 pounds. She looks at least 15 years younger than she is, and she walks and acts younger than most people less than half her age. By the way, the best way to prevent osteoporosis is by strengthening the bones through weight training.

In the following chapters, you will learn that all carbohydrates are not created equal. You'll learn the amount of carbohydrates you need and about the glycemic scale which will indicate when to eat what type of carbohydrates. Also, you'll learn how much fiber to consume to stay healthy and to get leaner. You will learn that all fats are not created equal. You will be able to tell the difference between saturated and monounsaturated fats, essential fatty acids, how much fat you need, and what sources of fats are the healthiest and least healthy. You'll learn what type of protein and how much you need for your particular size, how many meals to eat, and how much water to drink, which foods to avoid permanently, and which foods to add to your current nutritional program as well as information about antioxidant vitamin supplementation and other issues that will help you live younger and longer. There are several different diets in this book to get you to the size and shape you want to be and then to a permanent, healthy eating life-style that will keep you there. You will be heart healthy, lean on the inside and outside for the rest of your life.

As a personal trainer, I often take new clients that are 50 years old or older. At the very beginning, I tell them they are only at the halfway mark of their life and the next 50 years are determined by the change in habits, a successful nutrition program, and regular exercise, both anaerobic and aerobic to keep the heart in good shape as well as all the muscles throughout the body strong, toned, and limber. They have an opportunity to help determine not only the quantity of years, but the quality of life in the years to come. And you too, by putting to practice the secrets and knowledge in this book, can greatly enhance the way you feel about yourself, the way others view you, and your overall physical health and vitality.

Don't feel like you have to change everything overnight! Be quick to congratulate yourself when you implement a new habit and stick with it replacing old bad habits. Remember, either your habits are a slave to you, or you are a slave to them. I recommend that you develop good habits and let them work for you. Also keep in mind that success by the inch is a cinch, but by the yard is hard. Don't expect an instant miracle. I have people who come to me and say "My class reunion is in three weeks. I've got to drop 50 pounds—what can I do?" Well, unless you want to get a leg amputated, to be honest, there's not a lot you can do. However, a reasonable goal will drop ten pounds of fat per month while maintaining muscle, depending on the amount of fat you currently have. So relax, read, and incorporate the principles that you learn into your daily life. You will be glad that you did. So will your family and friends. Good luck and God bless you in your effort to become a new you and the best that you can be.

Sumo Syndrome—Could this be you?

I am about to tell you how to get big—sumo wrestler style! You're probably saying, "This is exactly what I don't want to do!" However, this is the way that many Americans eat! As a matter of fact, Americans are the most over fat people of any country in the world. Obesity is the second highest cause of preventable death in the United States. We are in the midst of an obesity epidemic!

The physiological purpose and function for fat is to store excess glucose. The average fat cell size is 0.5 microns. However, if you work at it, you can get it four times that size.

The way that sumo wrestlers get so huge is by fasting pretty much all day until the evening. Then they eat and because they are so hungry by this time, they literally gorge. They eat fast. When your hypothalamus, which produces your hunger hormones, kicks in, you have no willpower. If you eat fast, when your brain begins to send signals that you are full, you are already over full by the time you feel these signals. Sumo wrestlers don't eat until they are famished. They gorge on high fat, high carbohydrate meals, consuming thousands of calories at one sitting. Immediately upon eating, they roll over and go to sleep or rest.

Now how many people do you know who say they don't eat breakfast because they get hungry two or three hours later. They may skip lunch, come home, eat like there is no tomorrow, go to the easy chair, sit in front of the television, and go to sleep. Then they wonder why they can't lose weight eating just one meal a day.

Obviously, this is not what they are after. In the following chapters, you are going to be encouraged to eat six times a day. All of these tips are designed to help you lose on a consistent basis until you get to where you want to go. At the end of the book, there is a chapter on measuring and charting your success. However, weight management boils down to "waist management." Get a tape measure and measure the largest part of your waist. That's what we want to reduce.

A reasonable goal, since people of all sizes are using these proven methods, will vary individually. A good rule of thumb is to lose 1% of your start weight per week. This allows you to lose fat, but keep or even gain muscle if you follow the exercise routine given later. A three hundred and fifty pound person could anticipate losing 3^1/$_2$ pounds per week; a one hundred and eighty pound person could look at losing 1.8 pounds per week. Another reasonable goal would be to lose 10% of your start weight in the first 3-6 months. Remember, it's changing your behavior (your eating patterns and your exercise patterns) that you want to focus on, not the scale. These numbers are merely guidelines.

Rather than doing it "sumo style," you want to eat the majority of your calories during the day, beginning with an adequate breakfast that is high in fiber. This will cause you to burn an extra 200 calories. Plus, bran eaters eat less later in the day.

Let me explain how eating breakfast causes you to burn more calories. Your BMR (Basal Metabolic Rate) is the rate at which you burn calories while resting. This is also referred to as resting energy expenditure. This is where 70% of your calories are consumed. By the way, if you have been on the yo-yo syndrome where you have gained weight and lost weight and gained weight and lost weight, then it may take a while for your BMR to get readjusted. But as you focus on your new behavior, this will happen so that you begin to burn more calories at rest.

I recommend you exercise for at least 20 minutes once every 12 hours. For instance, 20 minutes at 6:00 a.m. and at least 20 minutes at 6:00 p.m. Twenty percent of your calories are burned during active energy expenditures, or during your exercise program. Ten percent (and this is where the eating six meals per day comes in) of your calories burned are referred to as TEE or thermic energy expenditure. This is where the body has to heat up to digest the food. So if you only eat once or twice a day, you're only taking advantage of that time once or twice a day. However, if you eat six times a day, then every time you eat your thermic energy expenditure kicks in and you can burn as much as 200 calories just through digesting a small meal.

Through eating small meals, there is very little excess food to be stored in fat cells. Also keep in mind that exercise is cumulative. So, develop habits such as taking the stairs instead of the elevator and parking farther away from the grocery store so you have to walk farther. Little things like that throughout the day and evening will cause you to burn more calories.

Do you realize that there are ¹/₃ more obese people today than there were 10 years ago? A big part of this is due to the fact that your parents burned, on the average, 500 calories more per day than you do. Just stop and think. Ten years ago, not everybody had a remote control television. They actually had to get up and change the channel. Twenty years ago, we drove stick shifts and had to roll the window down rather than push buttons. As we access more conveniences, we also burn fewer calories, so keep that in mind!

Also keep in mind that the sumo wrestler rolls over and rests as soon as he completes his gorging. Unlike the sumo wrestlers, you also need to eat slower so your brain can send you messages that enough is enough. That is part of the hormone process. Again, people who eat breakfast tend to eat smaller dinners.

What about genetics?

All of us have a genetically predisposed body type. Physiologists years ago referred to this as somatotype with three basic types: ectomorphic (people who tend to be tall and thin and generally have a difficult time gaining weight), mesomorphic (people who tend to be shorter and more muscular), and endomorphic (people who tend to be of medium height and plump). People are rated on a scale of 1-7 and all of us have some of each of these three body types, generally leaning more toward one than the other. The sex hormones, testosterone and estrogen, tend to make us more muscular or less muscular. The male hormones tend to cause us to lose fat. Therefore, there are some genetic predispositions. Two people who expend the same amount of calories sitting side by side, eating the same amount of food, can have different results. This is a direct result of inherited metabolism or genetic structure.

However, all of us can succeed in reshaping our bodies. Very few people have hormonal deficiencies enough to prevent them from losing fat. If you feel like you may be in this category, then I would suggest a good physical with a thorough blood workup, checking levels such as sex hormones, growth hormone, thyroid hormone, glucose tolerance, etc. In some cases, especially in middle aged and older people, hormone replacement therapy is becoming more common in both women and men. There are a number of physicians who will prescribe different types of hormones such as growth hormone, testosterone, thyroid hormone, etc., and in some cases this will enhance weight loss and muscle gain.

On the other hand, before we blame everything on our parents and the genes that we inherited, I would like to cite for you a study done on the Pima Indians. The American Pima Indians who live in the western United States are 100% overweight with a 97% diabetes rate. In Mexico their genetic twin Pima Indians have zero obesity and lower than average population diabetic rate. What is the difference? The American Pima Indians all have televisions with remote controls, drink a lot of alcohol, eat a lot of high fat, high carbohydrate foods and do very little in the way of physical activity.

On the other hand, the Mexican Pima Indians are poor. They basically farm for their living, eat high fiber, low fat foods, and burn a lot of calories in their daily activities. Therefore even though these two different groups are genetically identical, the socialization and the habits make all the difference.

If you have ever seen any pictures of a prison camp where people are starved, you will see people there of all genetic structures, but you won't see any obese people. If you show up for a marathon race, you will see people of all genetic propensities, but you will not find one single person who is obese.

Once again, we can all win, but it depends on a healthy life-style and avoiding the "Sumo Syndrome" and developing the life-style that you are going to read about in the coming chapters.

We have two other facts to discuss. If you are obese, (by the way, to find out if you are obese or not, look at the BMI chart at the end of the book and find yourself on the scale), realize that 1) You should view obesity as a chronic illness that needs continuous treatment. That is life-style, habitual, healthy living. Also realize that 2) The biggest medical gains are found in the first 10% of your fat loss. This is good news because fairly quickly in your fat loss program, you will begin to feel better, which itself is an intrinsic reward.

MR. MUSCLE
(Dr. Tom Owen)

- **World Strength Tour**

- **USA, Canada, Africa, Europe, Great Britain and the Orient and numerous national and international shows**

- **Featured on Spectacular World of Guinness, That's Incredible, FOX network's WOW-III (The World's Most Awesome Acts), Las Vegas, Live on the Jay Leno Show, The Crook & Chase Show In Hollywood, Viva Variety on Comedy Central, and hundreds of other shows, all over the world.**

This is a current photograph of Tom at a much leaner bodyweight of 235 lbs., with very little strength loss in the process!

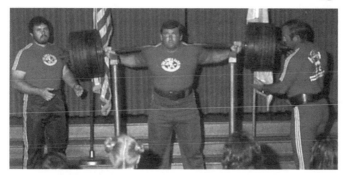

Tom at a bodyweight of 300 lbs., shown squatting over 700 lbs. for repetitions at an exhibition.

Chapter Two

LIFELONG FITNESS: PSYCHOLOGICAL ASPECTS

Physical Exercise Improves Mental Health— The Upward Spiral

Many studies have documented the fact that physical exercise relieves emotional stress. We live in a very stressful society. One of the main reasons I work out every day is for my psychological well-being.

While in graduate school, I researched an Auburn University study of 12 adolescents who exhibited problem behavior. These 12 teens enrolled in a daily exercise program that included cardiovascular and skeletal muscle strengthening exercises. During the study period, the teenagers had their physical fitness levels and their self-esteem levels tested. The conclusion of the study was that as the subjects' physical fitness level rose, so did their self-esteem! They began to feel better about themselves.

Adults don't differ much from adolescents. We hope that as adults we have a high level of maturity, but much of our self-esteem (or lack of it) is carried over from our childhood.

Exercise accomplishes several things. When we exercise, we feel invigorated physically. All of our systems are stimulated. We also feel emotionally energized. This is due in part to our feeling that we are doing something good for ourselves. Emotional energy is related to the release of endorphins that occurs when we exercise. Endorphins are chemicals produced by the brain that give us a general feeling of well-being. They tend to act as a pain reliever—physically and emotionally.

Psychology goes through fads, just as any other discipline. In the 1970's some psychologists propagated the ideology that if you were angry, you should hit a punching bag. Today, most psychologists feel this is counterproductive. Present day psychology teaches us that controlling our emotions is much healthier than unleashing them through screaming, kicking, etc.

However, the benefit of physical activity in alleviating emotional tension is well documented. Physical stress (through exercise instead of destructive behavior) does help to alleviate emotional stress.

I've seen many examples of the value of physical activity improving emotional outlook. One experience left an important lasting impression on me. During work on my master's degree and internship for my Ed.S., I worked in two psychiatric units—one for adults and one for adolescents. Some patients were suicidal, extremely depressed, and out of touch with reality. Some were involved in exercise, while others were not. The patients who exercised tended to heal much more quickly than those who remained dormant.

Albert Ellis, the founder of Rational-Emotive Therapy, made a very important observation. He discovered that a depressed patient who asserts himself can overcome the depression more readily than the passive patient. I maintain that when you assert yourself physically, you are actively putting yourself back in control of your situation.

Often, depression comes as a result of helplessness—a feeling of being out of control. Exercise helps you gain that control, which in turn helps you feel more complete with greater self-esteem. When you begin to see and feel the good results of regular exercise combined with correct eating, your efforts are reinforced. This helps you feel better about yourself. Feeling better encourages more regular exercise and continued good eating habits. So you begin an upward spiral toward general well-being, instead of a downward spiral where things seem only to get worse.

Sometimes I think the psychological benefits to exercise may be even greater than the physical benefits. And as you'll see later in this book, exercise does not have to hurt to work. Pick something you can enjoy and live with!

Psychological Aspects of Weight Loss and Control—God Does Not Make Any Junk

Physical exercise is good for your physique, but how does

body weight interact with your mental state? Take a minute to be introspective. Look inside and ask yourself, "What really is the problem that causes me to put on these extra pounds?" Granted, some of the reasons may be genetic. We all have different traits, and some of us gain fat cells more easily than others. However, all of us can succeed in shedding unwanted pounds—all of us!

Over the years, as a psychological therapist, a licensed professional counselor, and a personal fitness trainer, I have talked to many people who wanted to lose weight. Some people eat when they are happy since during their childhood each family celebration and outing centered around lots of sweets and fattening things to eat. Some people eat because they are angry, anxious, or depressed. For this group, eating feeds that downward spiral that causes them to feel even worse about themselves. Some people eat out of boredom or because they are nervous. Let's take a look at these negative emotions and habits that work against us.

It is imperative, I believe, to reinforce and elevate ourselves with positive thought. MAINTAIN A POSITIVE OUTLOOK. I believe that God is the Author of positive thinking. Philippians 4:8-9 says to think on those things that are lovely, pure, right, and good, and the peace of God shall be with us. Positive thinking is not the result of new-wave psychology or motivational speakers. It is God's plan for us to hold a positive perspective and outlook.

Psychologists use a term called "self talk." In Psalm 42, the psalmist says, "O my soul, why doest thou despair within me?" The psalmist is talking to himself here and asking why he says negative things to himself. We need to refrain from talking to ourselves in negative terms. Be good to yourself and talk to yourself in uplifting, positive terms.

Ninety percent of us perceive ourselves in a negative vein, at least part of the time. We don't like ourselves for any one of a number of reasons. We're too fat, too short, too shy, too pushy, not smart enough, or too poor. We've got lots of negative baggage that weighs us down. We subconsciously think, "I'm not worthy, so I'll just continue to punish myself. I'll eat and stay fat."

I want to challenge you to look at yourself as being OK already. I want you to feel worthy and acceptable, and because you're OK, you ought to get in shape. You deserve to feel better! Think about when you go to the beach—how good *you* will feel about yourself. Think about the possibility of a longer life, and the greater energy you'll have to live life to its fullest. Think about those good thoughts, and not the negative thoughts that come with self-denial. This helps keep you focused on your goal, which will help you succeed.

While your thoughts and focus are of utmost importance, you can also use some common sense along the way. For instance, for social functions, try filling up on low-calorie foods beforehand. Then you won't have to contend with true physical hunger, which may cause you to focus on the food in spite of your strong desire to look ahead in a positive way.

Avoid the P.O.M.S. (Poor Ole' Me Syndrome). This is a term I coined in graduate school. Instead of feeling sorry for yourself when you don't make your goal, focus on your behavior rather than focusing on how many pounds you've lost, let the success itself be the behavior changes that you have accomplished. This can include changing your eating habits, your exercise habits, and so on. Remember that success is a journey, not a destination. Enjoy your journey every step of the way!

Habits—Make Them Work For You

Habits can either work for you or against you. If you're overweight, no doubt you're eating when you're not truly hungry. Overeating has become a habit—in this case one that's working against you. The answer is to change your habit. Get the habit to work for you. This is particularly important after you have lost weight. Habits play a vital role in maintaining your weight.

Your habits were not developed in one day, and they won't change in one day. However, modern psychology teaches us that if we do the same thing 21 days in a row, we can incorporate that into our personality as a new habit. You will find that if you can discipline yourself for a brief period of time, then every day it gets a little easier. The toughest day for the drug addict during his rehabilitation is the first day. The second day is not quite as bad, and the third day is better. A lot of staying in shape is merely adapting some new life-style habits that help you have more energy, more enthusiasm, and increased health and vigor.

Formerly, when I would stop to get gasoline, I would automatically buy a candy bar also. I no longer do that. Before, it was almost an unconscious habit. Now, I have made it a habit not to do that. It took a little while to break that habit, but now I no longer associate buying gas with buying a candy bar.

Neurolinguistic programming is a new form of psychology that deals with a highly refined sense of "association," or associating certain events with other events. For example: associating going to a movie with eating popcorn. When we make a conscious effort to change a habit, such as going to five movies in a row without eating popcorn, then your new behavior can become a habitual act. The original association of movie and popcorn loses its strength and eventually is broken completely.

Just like the movie-popcorn example, you can change habits that are causing you to overeat. Start by taking time to write down all the things that you associate with food. Do it now. After completing this list, look at the types of food that you associate with various events. There is a two-step, sure-fire way to change those habits: (1) Do that event five times in a row without eating anything—quitting "cold turkey." (2) Eat a different food, one that is low fat and healthy, in its place at the event—five times in a row.

You can also combine steps 1 and 2 for events that don't take place frequently. The next time you go to a party, have fun, enjoy yourself, but munch on high-fiber and low-calorie foods, such as carrot sticks or celery.

Remember to focus on the long-term benefits and not the food. Then do it again at your next social event. Wow! You have just succeeded in substituting a habit that worked against you for a habit that works for you. Continue to do this for a few more parties, and you'll have a habit that will serve you well for the rest of your life. Congratulate yourself now for determining to do this. Feel good about your small successes, and remember:

SUCCESS BY THE INCH IS A CINCH—
BY THE YARD IS HARD!

The longer you deny a craving, the weaker it gets and the stronger you get!

Lighten Up!

Things are seldom as bad as we make them out to be.

A questionnaire was given to a group of sharp senior citizens, all of whom were past retirement age. They were asked if they had their lives to live over again, what three things would they do differently. Here are their responses: (1) Don't take myself so seriously. (2) Laugh more. (3) Don't make big problems out of little problems.

So often we tend to make mountains out of molehills. We tend to do what I term "awfulize" the situation. We look at it and immediately label it as being absolutely awful, horrible, terrible. Well, occasionally we are all slapped in the face by some of life's harsh realities. However, I am a big believer in the fact that your attitude in life is controlled by only 10% of what happens to you, and 90% by the way you react to it.

Albert Ellis, the founder of Rational-Emotive Therapy, uses a diagram that I would like to explain to you. It is his contention that we don't have to accept the initial feelings or responses that come from life's situations. For instance, in his diagram are three phases: (1) The activating event; (2) The way you perceive that event; (3) The emotional outcome of that event. For example: (1) Someone slaps you in the face (figuratively); (2) You believe that it is horrible that someone slapped you in the face; (3) You are mad that someone slapped you in the face.

You can change the cycle. Why let an outside event cause destructive stress and possibly ruin your day? Try this instead: (1) Someone slaps you in the face; (2) You believe it could have been worse: you could have just been hit by a car! (3) Accept what happened, shake it off, and go on with your business without being *full* of negative emotion.

How does this relate to weight-loss and weight-control? When we miss our goal, we think it's awful and we begin to get really down on ourselves. The old downward spiral begins, which may end in another diet failure. Instead, next time say: "Yes, it was a mistake but it was not awful! I'm going to pick up here and start all over again." This way, you get out of the downward syndrome of saying to yourself that you're a failure, so why not be fat—that's all you deserve. Instead, you shake it off and try again with a positive, upbeat attitude.

Your attitude toward yourself and life in general is important since you may be eating because you're depressed. By changing your attitude in a positive, upbeat way, you avoid the depression and the overeating that only makes you feel worse. So the next time you feel bad—CHALLENGE that feeling. Remember, we cannot control the situations around us, but we can control the way we react to them.

It is not acceptable to say that someone really made you mad. Don't give someone that power. Only you have the power to decide how you feel. Don't allow outside circumstances to control your attitudes. Much of life is an attitude, and you can be in control of the way you feel regardless of your circumstances, regardless of those around you. DON'T ALLOW YOURSELF TO BE DEFEATED BY YOUR OWN NEGATIVE THOUGHTS.

Of course, there will still be times when you feel grief, disappointment, or sadness. You need to learn other ways to handle these feelings besides overeating. Read an encouraging book, talk to a friend, or take a brisk walk. Do something constructive, such as helping someone else, ventilating your feelings, or asserting yourself. Positive action can give you that little spark you need to help turn things around! Remember, you can control your eating with a positive attitude and by taking your focus away from food!

Get Some Help—Letter of Support

You can lose weight and maintain a trim healthy body all on your own. But why not get all the help you can? If you are beginning a weight-loss and weight-control program, you might find the following letter (or one similar to it) an asset in your quest to shape up and have a healthier lifestyle.

Dear Spouse, Child, Parent, or Friend:

I have decided to lose weight and get into better shape, and then to stay in shape. I need your help and support in doing this.

I am going to change my eating and drinking habits. This is really important to me, and I really want to succeed. Your encouragement and understanding will mean a great deal to me.

There will be times I will be grouchy or irritable because I feel hungry. Please bear with me during these times. It will be worth it—I assure you!

Thank you for your support and help during the weeks and months to come.

Chapter Three

HEALTHY EATING

All Carbs Are NOT Created Equal...

First of all, let me explain that almost all foods contain carbohydrates. The only foods that don't are meats, some cheeses, and eggs. In this chapter, we will focus largely on the glycemic index, which is included on page 28. The higher numbers on the glycemic index simply indicates how quickly the food turns into glucose in your system. Therefore, on a scale from 1 to 100, anything above 50 or 60 would be considered high glycemic index carbohydrates. Below 35 would be considered low glycemic index carbohydrates, which convert much more slowly to glucose.

Why is this important? Because of two reasons. First, while the caloric content may be virtually the same as a high glycemic and a low glycemic food, there is a double whammy associated with higher glycemic index carbohydrates. Because a substance such as sugar candy converts so quickly to glucose, if you consume enough of this (several hundred calories or more) at one time, your blood sugar levels would rise. This stimulates your pancreas to produce more insulin, which is good if you have just finished a hard workout, but that is the *only* time it is good. The rest of the day, when insulin is secreted, its job is to force your blood sugar level back to normal.

Insulin is one of the most powerful hormones in the body. If you have just worked out, the insulin will force the glucose into the hungry muscle cells restoring the glycogen content. However, if your muscle cells are not hungry or depleted then it will be stored as fat wherever you are genetically predisposed to carry additional adipose tissue (fat). That's why I ask, "Do you like this food enough to wear it?" Because when you consume high glycemic index carbohydrates, especially along with fat calories, your body very quickly will convert that to stored energy and you *will* wear it. On the other hand, carbohydrates such as black-eyed peas, soybeans, etc., are converted very slowly to glucose, therefore not stimulating a blood sugar level rise and allowing the carbohydrates to be used more as prolonged energy. This would be a good pre-workout meal.

Traditionally, people have thought that it was good to eat candy or high glycemic carbohydrates prior to a workout to be used as fuel. However, just the opposite is true. An hour or so before you work out, it's better to consume lower glycemic carbohydrates and then small amounts of higher glycemic index carbohydrates immediately after working out. In essence, the only time you ever want high glycemic carbohydrates is within an hour after you have completed your workout. Otherwise, that same energy that would have been used to replenish muscle glycogen will now be used to fatten fat cells.

As a rule, carbohydrates that are high in fiber, such as beans, are lower on the glycemic scale. Also carbohydrates, when mixed with fats such as ice cream, surprisingly are also lower on the glycemic scale. This is why I never recommend that people drink fruit juices, because, many of them are laden with sugar. Natural fruit juice has the fiber taken out of it and as a result is higher glycemically than the actual fruit itself. As a matter of fact, I recommend that you consume no beverages with calories other than skim milk and/or protein drinks.

The traditional steak and potato diet that a lot of Americans are on is an ideal way to gain fat as well as clog up your arteries. A white baked potato is at the very top of the glycemic index, whereas a good substitute for that would be a sweet potato which is lower. Apples are also low and very healthy. I mentioned the term "carbohydrate sensitive." This can better be described as "insulin sensitivity." Depending on the extent of insulin resistance, serum glucose and serum insulin can rise causing the increased conversion of glucose to fat via the liver. If hepatic insulin resistance exists, the increased conversion is via a mechanism that involves the arterial walls. Individuals with varying degrees of insulin resistance, which limits the ability to use carbohydrates more efficiently, can benefit from consuming lower glycemic carbohydrates simply because they digest more slowly. This slows the addition of glucose, giving the body more time to use the carbohydrates for energy, rather than be stored as fat. I believe your diet eventually should have approximately 40% carbohydrates, simply because that's where all fiber is derived. Again, these carbs should be on the lower end of the glycemic scale.

I have been exercising for 30 years and during the 1990's it became very important for me to stay lean as a competitive Master's Bodybuilder. Because I have learned how to manipulate my diet, which in turn manipulates my metabolism, it's easier for me to stay lean now than it ever has been, simply through changing my habits. One main factor is avoiding foods that turn to glucose too quickly. The word *glycemic* is easily translated as "blood sugar response" and comes from the word *glycemia* which is defined as "the presence of glucose in the blood." It is the amount of this glucose that is the main concern, especially as to how quickly the levels rise which again is directly related to the Glycemic Index. So use the following index as a guide that will help you determine how to get all the fiber you need through carbohydrates, but will help you avoid the insulin response as a result of eating too much high glycemic carbohydrates at any one time. If you have to have something that's high on the glycemic scale, limit it to 100 calories (or 25 grams) and at the same time eat another food with fat to help lower your index. A side benefit from this is that you will not have the up and down of the blood sugar levels as you would from eating high glycemic carbohydrates. This causes elevated blood sugar levels and then the insulin response causes lowered blood sugar level, making you again to be hungry for more high glycemic carbohydrates. Eating lower glycemic carbohydrates will help level out your blood sugar levels and ease those hunger pains.

The Glycemic Index (GI) value of foods is adjusted propor-
tionately so that the GI of white bread = 100 (* = foods converted where necessary from glucose base = 100 by multiplying by 1.38).

Glycemic Index (By Food Groups)

Breads

Rye		
Crispbread	95	
Whole meal	89	
Whole grain,		
i.e., pumpernickel	68	
Wheat		
White	100	
Whole meal	100	

Pasta

Macaroni	
White, boiled 5 min.	64
Spaghetti	
Brown, boiled 15 min.	61
White, boiled 15 min.	61
White, boiled 5 min.	45
Protein enriched	38
Star pasta	
White, boiled 5 min.	54

Tortilla

Corn	100*

Cereal grains

Barley (pearled)	31
Buckwheat	74
Bulgur	65
Millet	103
Rice	
Brown	81
Instant, boiled 1 min.	65
Instant, boiled 6 min.	121
Polished, boiled 5 min.	58
Polished, boiled 15 min.	79
Parboiled, boiled 5 min.	54
Parboiled, boiled 25 min.	65
Rye kernels	47
Sweet corn	80
Wheat kernels	63

Breakfast cereals

All Bran	74
Cornflakes	115
Muesli	96
Porridge oats	87
Puffed rice	132
Shredded wheat	97
Weetabix	109

Cookies

Digestive	82
Oatmeal	78
Rich tea	80
Plain crackers	
(water biscuits)	91
Ryvita	95
Pastry	81*
Sponge cake	63*

Root vegetables

Beetroot	88*
Carrots	117*
Parsnips	134*
Potato	
Instant	118
Mashed	100
New, boiled	80
Russet, baked	128
Sweet	70
Rutabaga (Swede)	99*
Yam	74

Legumes

Baked beans (canned)	60
Bengal gram dal	12
Black beans	43*
Black-eyed peas	46*
Brown beans	54*
Broad beans (Fava beans)	109*
Butter beans	46
Chick peas (Garbanzo)	49

Green peas		Plum	34
Dried	50	Raisins	88*
Frozen	65	**Sugars**	
Marrowfat	65*	Fructose	31
Haricot (white) beans	57	Glucose	138
Kidney beans	45	Honey	126
Lima beans	50*	Maltose	152
Red lentils	37	Sucrose	89
Soy beans		**Snack foods**	
Dried	20	Corn chips	99
Canned	22	Potato chips	77
Fruit		Peanuts	15
Apricots, dried	46	Mars Bar	94*
Apricots, canned	91	**Dairy products**	
Apple	53	Ice cream	52
Apple juice	59	Skim milk	46
Banana	84	Whole milk	49
Fruit cocktail	79	2% milk	48*
Grapes	62	Yogurt	52
Grapefruit juice	69	**Miscellaneous**	
Orange	59	Fish fingers	52*
Orange juice	67	Lucozade	131*
Peaches	40	Nopal (prickly pear)	10*
Peaches, canned	74	Sausages	39*
Pears	58	Tomato soup	52*
Pears, canned	63		
Pineapple juice	66		

Glycemic Index (High to Low)

		109	Weetabix
		109	Broad beans (Fava beans)
152	Maltose	103	Millet
138	Glucose	100	Tortilla, corn
134	Cooked parsnips	100	Potato, mashed
132	Puffed rice	100	Bread, wheat, whole meal
131	Lucozade	100	Bread, wheat, white
128	Potato, Russet, baked	99	Rutabaga (Swede)
126	Honey	99	Corn chips
121	Rice, instant, boiled 6 min.	97	Shredded wheat
118	Potato, instant	96	Muesli
117	Cooked carrots	95	Cookies, Ryvita
115	Cornflakes	95	Bread, rye, crispbread

GI-based list (continued):

94	Mars Bar	61	Spaghetti, brown, boiled 15 min.
91	Cookies, plain crackers	60	Baked beans (canned)
91	Apricots, canned	59	Orange
89	Sucrose	59	Apple juice
89	Bread, rye, whole meal	58	Rice, polished, boiled 5 min.
88	Raisins	58	Pears
88	Beetroot	57	Haricot (white) beans
87	Porridge oats	54	Rice, parboiled, boiled 5 min.
84	Banana	54	Pasta, star white, boiled 5 min.
82	Cookies, digestive	54	Brown beans
81	Rice, brown	53	Apple
81	Pastry	52	Yogurt
80	Sweet corn	52	Tomato soup
80	Potato, new, boiled	52	Ice cream
80	Cookies, rich tea	52	Fish fingers
79	Rice, polished, boiled 15 min.	50	Lima beans
79	Fruit cocktail	50	Green peas, dried
78	Cookies, oatmeal	49	Whole milk
77	Potato chips	49	Chick peas (Garbanzo)
74	Yam	48	2% milk
74	Peaches, canned	47	Rye kernels
74	Buckwheat	46	Skim milk
74	All Bran	46	Butter beans
70	Potato, sweet	46	Blackeye peas
69	Grapefruit juice	46	Apricots, dried
68	Bread, rye pumpernickel	45	Spaghetti, white, boiled 5 min.
67	Orange juice	45	Kidney beans
66	Pineapple juice	43	Black beans
65	Rice, parboiled, boiled 25 min.	40	Peaches
65	Rice, instant, boiled 1 min.	39	Sausages
65	Green peas, marrowfat	38	Pasta, spaghetti, protein enriched
65	Green peas, frozen	37	Red lentils
65	Bulgur	34	Plum
64	Macaroni, white, boiled 5 min	31	Fructose
63	Wheat kernels	31	Barley (pearled)
63	Sponge cake	22	Soy beans, canned
63	Pears, canned	20	Soy beans, dried
62	Grapes	15	Peanuts
61	Spaghetti, white, boiled 15 min.	12	Bengal gram dal
		10	Nopal (prickly pear)

...Neither Are Fats and Proteins Created Equal.

Fats are divided by type into saturated, monounsaturated, and polyunsaturated. This is a chemical distinction based on the number of hydrogen atoms that are attached to the fatty acid's carbon chain. If all the available space is occupied by hydrogen, the fatty acid is called a saturated fatty acid. The fatty acid is unsaturated if less than the maximum number of hydrogen atoms are attached. If there is one double bond in the fatty acid, it is called a *mono*unsaturated fatty acid. If there is more than one double bond, it is called a *poly*unsaturated fatty acid.

The degree of saturation influences the melting point of the fatty acid. Saturated fats have a high melting point and are solid at room temperature. The fat that is visible in beef is due to the high content of saturated fat. Monounsaturated fats are typically liquid, but will become cloudy when placed in the refrigerator. Polyunsaturated fats stay liquid even in the cold because their melting point is lower than monounsaturated fats. Cooking oils (which are natural mixtures of various fatty acids) are mostly monounsaturated and/or polyunsaturated fatty acids. Olive oil is a good example of mostly monounsaturated fatty acids, while canola oil has considerable polyunsaturated fatty acids.

A very important reason to consider which dietary fats to include in your daily diet is the reduction of the risk or incidence of cardiovascular disease. Paying attention to fat composition (by increasing consumption of monounsaturated fats at the expense of saturated fat, while maintaining adequate polyunsaturated intake [10% of total calories]), results in better lipid profiles reflected in LDL and HDL levels and greater cardiovascular risk reduction. With more attention payed towards the fat composition, higher levels of fat in the diet can be tolerated and result in overall better health.

A subset of dietary fatty acids—linoleic acid and linolenic acid (also known as omega-6 and omega-3, respectively)—are essential to consume. The body requires fat to function properly, and these polyunsaturated fatty acids are two types that our bodies cannot manufacture by itself and they must therefore be obtained from your diet.

Another function of fat is as a source of energy. Fatty acids are very calorically dense with 9 calories per gram of fat. Carbohydrates and proteins are only 4 calories per gram. In addition, the body has limited ability to store carbohydrate (in the form of glycogen) because it requires a lot of supporting water to maintain the structure. In fact, the average person carries around about 1 pound of glycogen with an additional 4 pounds of water. This is why calorie restricted diets are diuretic in nature for the first few days; as the glycogen is used up (and not replaced), the water is lost along with it. Muscle tissue is 72% water by weight, so a little loss of muscle protein, causes a large loss of total weight. Alternatively, fat can be efficiently stored (much to the dismay of dieters). Because of its chemical structure, fat doesn't require a lot of water to sustain it. In adipose tissue (the storage form of fat), about 85% of the total weight is actual fat. Thus, from the body's energy perspective, fat is the obvious choice as a storage form of excess energy.

Protein

Proteins are formed by linking amino acids together into chemical chains. There are 20 amino acids required by the body for proper function. Eight of these are called essential amino acids because the body is not able to synthesize them, and they must therefore be provided in your diet.

Proteins are classified as either complete or incomplete. A complete protein contains all of the essential amino acids, while an incomplete protein lacks one or more of the essential amino acids. Complete protein sources include whey, fish, poultry, eggs, milk and meat.

When participating in an exercise program, it is important to consume enough protein in your diet to promote muscle growth. As part of a good diet, you should seek to consume proteins which are of high quality. This means that the protein should be efficiently used by the body—that they should be of high bioavailability. Bioavailability is a measure of how much of the protein you eat is absorbed by your body.

The most accurate way of testing the bioavailability of proteins is the Biological Value (BV) method. The BV is calculated by dividing the total nitrogen retained from eating a protein by the total nitrogen absorbed from eating that same protein. That figure is multiplied by 100 to express the number as a percentage of nitrogen retention. The BV scores for different protein sources reveal exactly which proteins the body absorbs best. Higher numbers mean higher absorption. The following list indicates some common proteins and their BV's. Currently, whey protein isolate is at the top of the list, whereas vegetable sources tend to be at the lower end.

Dietary Protein Source	Biological Value
Whey Protein Isolate	159
Whey Protein Concentrate	104
Whole egg	100
Milk	91
Egg White	88
Chicken	79
Casein	77
Soy	74

Get Lean and Stay That Way!

When we talk about eating healthy, we not only want to end up with the fat off of the outside of your body, but out of the inside of your arteries as well. With some simple rules, we will give you a lifetime life-style nutritional guide to optimize your health and well-being. Before I go on, let me mention that later in the book, there are several specific diets that will help different people reach their short-term goals. However, long-term health is what we're after. It's not so important what you weigh four months from now as it is four years from now. So the following information is not considered a diet, it is considered a lifestyle change and most likely will require you to change some habits. However, you can do this!

<u>Rule number one</u> is going to be: **Don't eat anything fried.**

Now if you have grown up on fast food and fried food, this may hurt a little bit and your first reaction may be "I can't go without fried food!" Well, the fact is that you can and if you want to change, you will. Otherwise, doing the same habits, eating the same things, prepared the same way, will get you the same results. This will greatly jeopardize your health. Anytime you fry something, usually it's fried in a less than desirable oil or fat. You immediately double or even greatly multiply the caloric content of the food. For example, a potato itself is inherently not all that bad. However, if you fry it, it's full of grease. You could cut the same potato in the same size strips, bake them until they're crispy and get pretty much the same result. We must be crazy to take perfectly healthy foods such as lean meats like chicken and fish, batter them and fry them! If your only option for lean protein is to eat fried chicken, make sure that you peel all the skin off or find another option that's not fried. To sum it up, rule number one: Don't eat any fried foods!

<u>Rule number two:</u> **Stay away from sugar and processed foods that have sugar added.**

Keep in mind that even though a food may be low in fat, it

can still be full of calories from sugar that must be accounted for. As a matter of fact, the only diet where calories don't matter is the No Carbohydrate Diet mentioned later in the book. Otherwise, every calorie adds up as a measurement unit of energy: 1 pound = 3500 calories. So to put it very simply, to lose two pounds, a week you must burn an additional 500 calories and limit your intake by 500 calories per day. These thousand calories per day will equal a two-pound per week fat loss. For all the previously mentioned reasons, avoid sugar!

Rule number three: **Drink no calories other than protein drinks or skim milk.**

Here you might ask, "What about fruit juice?" Keep in mind that even though fruit juice itself can contain vitamins and is generally healthier than sugary cola type beverages, it's still calories and those calories, once again, must be accounted for. It just kills me to see someone drinking sweetened tea as it is made in the southern states rather than unsweetened tea with an artificial sweetener added. The taste is virtually the same, yet in each glassful you're excluding up to 200 calories. The same thing is true with diet colas versus sugary colas. A person could lose 15 pounds a year just by cutting out the sugar in beverages and drinking just minimal amounts. So don't take in those unnecessary calories when you can acquire a taste for sugar free diet beverages.

Rule number four: **Use skim dairy products only — not just non-fat milk, but non-fat yogurt, non-fat cheese, etc.**

Dairy products are rich in calcium and good quality protein, but the fat is not necessary. And don't be fooled by percentages. Be a label reader! When I suggest to people that they drink skim milk rather than whole milk, sometimes I'm countered with "Well, I drink 2% milk." Two percent sounds like a very low percentage, but when you compare the grams in 2% milk to that in skim milk, there is 600% more fat in 2% than there is in skim. So don't be misled by percentages. Always look at the grams as you read labels. Also, keep your saturated fat grams to a very minimum. Let your fats come from healthier sources such as olive oil, flaxseed oil, etc.

Where condiments are concerned, use only fat free. Fat free mayonnaise is fine but remember any white based salad dressing is going to be full of fat so be careful and avoid those hundreds of extra calories that come unnecessarily.

Rule number five: **Limit your intake of red meat to small quantities of only the leanest cuts with all visible fat trimmed.**

Rule number six: **Drink a minimum of 64 ounces of water per day on top of any other beverages you may drink.**

The way to figure your optimum amount of water needed is by multiplying your body weight by $^2/_3$ or 66%. In other words, if you weigh 200 pounds, then you need 132 ounces of water. Obviously, some of this water will come from diet beverages and any other liquids you drink, as well as from most fruits and vegetables because they are between 50 and 90% water.

Rule number seven: **Take in a minimum of 25 grams of fiber per day, both soluble and insoluble.**

This will be further discussed later in the chapter.

Rule number eight: **Choose low calorie, low fat EVERY-THING!**

No sugar should be added!

Rule number nine: **Take vitamin supplements, including an aspirin, everyday.**

This will be discussed more thoroughly later.

Finally, if all this has you feeling so deprived that you can't live with it, then plan on one day a week to eat whatever you want. However, you cannot do this on the No Carbohydrate Diet, which is discussed later on. If you do blow your diet, just get up, get over it, and get on with it. Don't beat yourself up! Everybody slips occasionally, but just get right back on the wagon and make these habits work for you. Follow these rules and you'll be healthier and happier.

As far as when to eat, my suggestion is to become a grazer and eat all throughout the day. First thing in the morning, begin your day with a healthy breakfast that would consist perhaps of a bowl of bran cereal, an egg, with two extra egg whites, 12 ounces of skim milk, and black coffee if you would like. Perhaps instead of the bran cereal, have two slices of forty-calorie whole-wheat toast, which will provide you with approximately the same amount of fiber. At 10:00 a.m., snack on either an apple or banana; both will provide you with approximately four grams of fiber and some mid-glycemic carbohydrates. Drink a large glass of water or perhaps a sandwich using fat free mayonnaise, mustard, a couple of slices of very low fat chicken or turkey, a slice of fat free cheese, and maybe a slice of tomato and lettuce. At lunch, a grilled chicken salad with olive oil and vinegar dressing would be good perhaps with a side order of black-eyed peas or pinto beans, and unsweetened iced tea. At 3:00 p.m. have another snack again, maybe a piece of fruit or a sandwich. Dinner would be perhaps a couple of vegetables, with 4-8 ounces of grilled chicken, fish, or sliced turkey. Finally have an evening or bedtime snack consisting of fat free, sugar free yogurt, a cup of diet popcorn, or even a bowl of bran cereal with skim milk and artificial sweetener.

By eating all day long, especially low glycemic carbohydrates, your sugar cravings will go away and the only hunger that you will feel will be psychological. You're certainly not depriving yourself and you are feeding your body maybe better than you ever have before.

Regarding alcohol, it retards the body's use of fat for energy, as well as being very calorie dense. So as far as getting weight off and keeping it off, alcohol will be a detriment. If you must drink, do so in moderation, and only on special occasions.

Calories—How many?

Everybody's metabolism is different. As a rule of thumb, I recommend that if you are a male and you weigh 250 pounds, but you would like to weigh 160 pounds, that you get approximately 1600 calories per day. That is roughly ten times multiplied by the amount that you would like to weigh at the end of your diet. For some people, this will work quickly; for some people this won't work at all, especially if you have been on severely restricted calorie diets previously then you may want to refer to one of the special diets in the back of this book. It has been shown, however, that calorie restriction can play a very useful part, not only in losing weight, but also in fighting disease and increasing longevity.

On the weight loss part of your healthy nutrition program, as you are restricting your calories to no more than ten times the amount that you want to end up weighing, keep in mind that it's actually better to vary that a little from one day to the next. For instance, if your desired weight is 160 pounds, on Monday you may want to eat 1600 calories. On Tuesday, you may want to eat 1800 calories and on Wednesday, you may want to reduce that to 1400 calories. I also want to recommend here again that if you can stimulate your metabolism by exercising every 12 hours for at least 20 minutes, for example a brisk walk in the morning and then a weight lifting session in the evening or vice versa. This will help keep your metabolism going and the frequent, smaller meals will also help keep your metabolism going. At this caloric intake, you should not go into what is called the starvation syndrome when your body tries to adjust to a severely restricted diet by slowing down its metabolism and conserving fat. Unfortunately, some people are far too efficient at conserving fat and it is more difficult for them to lose than it is for others. So you must continually "fool" the body. By eating six times a day, getting more than adequate nutrition and at the same time restricting calories, is the safest, healthiest way to get the weight off and keep it off. Once you reach the point where you want to be, then you can adjust your calories. When you reach your desired weight level, if it is 160 for example, once you reach 155 to 160, then you can gradually increase calories. But remember to eat primarily low glycemic carbohydrates. Again, get your fats from healthy sources and your proteins from lean sources.

As far as percentages of how much of which nutrient, I believe that if you are a hard training athlete, you need as much as one gram of protein per day per pound of body weight. In my case, I compete at bodybuilding competitions weighing 230 pounds with a body fat percentage of less than 5%. So I believe that I should get at least 230 grams of protein per day. If your lean body mass is 100 pounds, and you're lifting hard, you should also get 100 grams of protein per day. If you are not lifting really hard, then you can get by with as little as $1/2$ gram of protein per pound of lean body weight, but not less than that. If you deprive your body from protein from external sources, then it will get it internally, which will weaken your heart and other organs.

Your nutrients should fall somewhere in the guidelines of anywhere from 30-50% high quality lean protein, 30-40% carbohydrates and 20-30% fats from healthy sources, depending on the amount of exercise, etc.

Regarding fruits and vegetables, remember even though we do suggest vitamin supplementation, there are certain things that are found in fruits and vegetables that are not found in a vitamin pill, such as lycopene which is found in tomatoes, that can help protect men from prostate problems. Potassium, found in bananas, can help stabilize blood pressure. While some meal replacement food bars and nutritious drinks can be helpful, real food should be your primary source of calories for the vital nutrients, chemicals, and fiber that the fresh fruits and vegetables can provide, as well as a feeling of fullness and satisfaction.

Even though most of us do not want to be competitive bodybuilders, they are the leanest, most muscular athletes in the world and during competition season, it's rare to see a bodybuilder without a cooler in his hand where he has measured amounts of food that he will graze on all day long, such as pasta, chicken, or black-eyed peas and turkey. With things of this nature, he or she gets more than adequate nutrition, ample protein, carbohydrates and fats, but in very metered quantities and at specific times throughout the day.

What about workout meals?

To conclude, one meal that I want to stress that is very important is the post-workout meal. This is the time when you should have up to 50 grams of high glycemic carbohydrates along with 20 or more grams of easily digested, high quality protein enriched in the amino acid glutamine with potassium. Your muscles grow not while you are working out, but in between workouts and you have a window of opportunity right after you work out where your muscles are particularly hungry. During this time, the high glycemic carbohydrates will stimulate your pancreas to release insulin, which will then force the nutrients (the glycogen and the amino acids) into the muscle cells to begin immediately in facilitating the growth and restoration of the muscle cells. This is the one time of day that you do want to have the high glycemic carbohydrates. As far as pre-workout meals, I suggest lower glycemic carbohydrates that will provide the glycogen that you need to sustain the energy necessary for the workout.

Lowering Cholesterol

Oftentimes, people come to me saying "My doctor has told me that I have got to lower my cholesterol." First of all, of equal importance is not only the overall cholesterol number, but also the amount of HDL, LDL, and VLDL. High-density lipoproteins, HDL, are referred to as the "good guys"; low-density lipoproteins, LDL, are referred to as the "bad guys"; and very low-density lipoproteins, VLDL, are referred to as, you guessed it, "very bad guys."

The following steps will not only drastically help reduce cholesterol, but will actually help reverse the blockage that occurs when that cholesterol oxidizes on the inside of the artery and builds up the plaque, which can eventually completely occlude, or stop, the blood flow of that artery, leading to a stroke or heart attack.

Number one: **Eliminate the majority of saturated fat from your diet, which comes primarily from meat and dairy products.**

Number two: **Increase the healthy fats such as olive oil and flaxseed oil.**

Number three: **Increase the soluble fiber.** Soluble fiber such as oat bran, corn bran, pectin from apples, will help carry the cholesterol out of your system, taking it out of your body. Another good source of soluble fiber is psyllium, a popular fiber supplement that comes from the seeds of the plantago plant, a native to India and the Mediterranean area. It's used as a laxative in over-the-counter preparations and on a weight basis, soluble fiber makes up for about 75% of the psyllium seed as compared to the oat bran's 8% soluble fiber. Studies have reported that adding psyllium to the diet can help lower elevated blood cholesterol levels.

Number four: **Drink plenty of water.**

One time I actually lowered my cholesterol from the high 200's after being on a weight gain program to 99 through following these simple steps. So you want to make sure you eat two to three apples per day, a couple of bowls of corn or oat bran fiber cereal, as well as eliminating all cholesterol from your diet. If you follow the previous chapter, you pretty much would have done that anyway. You can make drastic changes quickly and that, coupled with aerobic and anaerobic exercise, can turn you into a different person.

You can actually raise the good kind of cholesterol, the

HDL, through aerobic exercise and you can help protect your arteries by taking in the antioxidant vitamins and minerals mentioned in Supplementation. Basically, 600 to 800 international units (IU) per day of Vitamin E, 15,000 IU's per day of beta-carotene, and 2000 milligrams (mgs) per day of Vitamin C, as well as an aspirin. This coupled with the fiber and the low cholesterol will get you amazing results in lowering your cholesterol. This can actually reverse the damage done by previous eating habits!

Heart Health

The heart is by far the most important muscle in the body. So keep these simple principles in mind to take care of your heart so it can take care of you.

Number one: Establish the nutritious, healthy lifetime eating program that has just been discussed.

Number two: Get enough sleep (7-8 hours per night).

Number three: Don't smoke. Over 50% of deaths due to preventable cause are attributed to cigarettes.

Number four: Avoid excess alcohol.

Number five: Make sure that you keep your blood pressure under control.

Number six: Avoid too much stress and remember that exercise is one of the best ways to alleviate emotional stress.

Number seven: Increase the High Density Protein (HDL), the "good guys" as mentioned before, in your diet.

Number eight: Get a good physical exam by a reputable physician, including a full blood profile.

As a final note, if you don't take responsibility and control of your health, then unfortunately, it will control you. It's a whole lot more fun to prevent a heart attack than rehabilitation if you happen to survive your first one. A lot of people use their first heart attack as a wake up call. That's not necessary. Heart disease kills more people than any other single illness.

Over 4000 Americans will suffer a heart attack *today*. Half of these victims had no warning. When questioned carefully, most people who suffer these attacks have continued deadly habits and ignored their body's danger signals for years. Whether you have had no sign of heart disease or even if you have already suffered a major heart attack, you can begin right now to protect yourself from the awful consequences of a lifestyle that leads to disaster. Take control, take responsibility and implement these changes.

Fiber-Important Additional Benefits

When most of us think of fiber, we imagine bran cereal. The fact that we need to eat fiber has been widely publicized. Let's see why we need fiber, and then recommend some excellent sources of fiber.

Fiber is a naturally occurring substance found in most plant foods. As these plant foods are eaten and digested, the fiber is separated from the other nutrients in the food. Fiber can be classified as either soluble or insoluble. Each type of fiber has benefits. Let's discuss them.

Soluble fiber is the type of fiber that is found in oat bran. Oat bran's recent claim to fame is that it lowers cholesterol. Foods that are good sources of soluble fiber are fruits, seeds, legumes (beans and peas), oats, and barley.

Insoluble fiber is found primarily as cellulose, which is undigestible by humans. This means it will pass through the digestive tract intact. This cellulose has a great affinity for water, which causes it to swell while in the digestive tract. This has two positive effects. First, it causes the sensation of fullness in the stomach, and second, it increases fecal volume. This results in decreased hunger and increased regularity. Foods that are high in insoluble fiber are wheat bran, beans, whole grains, fruits and vegetables.

Health benefits of fiber include:
- Improved weight management

- Decreased constipation
- Reduced blood cholesterol
- Decreased coronary artery disease
- Blood glucose and insulin regulation (diabetes control)
- Decreased chance of appendicitis
- Reduced chance of diverticulitis
- Reduced chance of colon cancer

The next big question is how much fiber should be consumed per day? Here again, reading labels and becoming familiar with the fiber content of foods is necessary. The recommended daily allowance for fiber is 25 or more grams per day. However, to experience the best health benefits, 50 to 60 grams should be consumed daily. This amount should not be consumed if you are pregnant or have certain mineral imbalances. You should gradually increase your fiber intake because gas and cramps can be a problem if fiber intake is increased too rapidly.

Fiber intake is only a small part of an overall sound eating plan, but its benefits can be tremendous. Here are some ways to *increase your fiber intake*:

- Eat whole-grain cereals each day. (The product should contain at least 5 grams dietary fiber per serving.)
- Eat whole wheat, cracked wheat, or stone-ground wheat bread.
- Eat popcorn instead of pretzels.
- Substitute brown rice for white rice.
- Six prunes have 10 grams of fiber, with no fat!
- Baked potato with skin is the veggie with the most fiber.

FIBER IN CEREALS

Cereal	Grams
All-Bran (Kellogg's)	8.6
All-Bran with extra Fiber (Kellogg's)	13.0
Bran Buds (Kellogg's)	7.7
Bran Chex (Post)	5.0

Corn Bran (Quaker)	5.9
Corn Flakes (Kellogg's)	trace
Cracklin' Oat Bran (Kellogg's)	4.1
Fiber One (General Mills)	12.0
40% Bran Flakes (All Brands)	4.3
Frosted Mini-Wheats (Kellogg's)	3.0
Fruit & Fiber (Post)	4.0
Fruitful Bran (Kellogg's)	4.0
Grape-Nuts (Post)	2.2
Natural Bran Flakes (Post)	5.0

Cereal	*Grams*
Nutri Grain (Kellogg's)	2.1
Oat Bran (1/3 cup)	4.2
Oatmeal (cooked)	trace
Oatmeal (uncooked)	1.0
100% Bran (Nabisco)	9.1
Product 19 (Nabisco)	trace
Raisin Bran (Kellogg's, Post)	2.9
Ralston Instant (Ralston)	3.3
Rice Krispies (Kellogg's)	trace
Shredded Wheat (Nabisco)	3.3
Shredded Wheat 'n Bran (Nabisco)	3.3
Total (General Mills)	2.5
Wheat Chex (Ralston)	2.5
Wheat Germ	5.5
Wheaten (Uhlmann)	4.0
Wheaties (General Mills)	2.5

WHERE TO FIND FIBER

Vegetables	Fiber Content (Gms)	Recommended Serving	Calories per serving
Asparagus	2.2	1 cup	50
Bean sprouts	3.9	1 cup	41
Beans			
Kidney	8.6	1 cup	225
Lima	12.6	1 cup	223

	Fiber Content (Gms)	Recommended Serving	Calories per serving
Pinto	12.7	1 cup	235
String	4.0	1 cup	19
Broccoli	5.4	1 cup	43
Brussels sprouts	6.7	1 cup	61
Cabbage	4.0	1 cup	31
Carrots	3.5	1 cup	47
Cauliflower	3.2	1 cup	34
Celery	1.9	1 cup	19
Corn	4.0	1 cup	160
Cucumber	2.0	1 cup	29
Eggplant	2.0	1 cup	22
Kale greens	4.3	1 cup	42
Onions	3.1	1 med	60
Parsnips	4.0	1 lrge	132
Peas	15.8	1 cup	179
Potatoes			
White	2.6	1 med	120
Sweet	3.0	1 med	140
Radish	.1	1 red	2
Zucchini	1.2	1 cup	18
Tomato	1.0	1 med	35
Turnip	1.2	1 cup	40
Fruit			
Apple	4.0	1 med	80
Apricots	.7	1 med	17
Banana	4.0	1 small	110
Blackberries	8.9	1 cup	75
Cherries	3.0	21	90
Grapefruit	5.0	1/2 avg	70
Grapes	1.0	1 1/2 cup	90
Orange	5.0	1 med	80
Peach	2.0	1 med	40
Pear	4.0	1 med	100

	Fiber Content (Gms)	Recommended Serving	Calories per serving
Pineapple	1.9	1 cup	76
Breads			
Bagel (Plain)	2.4	1 bagel	320
Cornbread	.6	1 slice	120
French (Pillsbury)	.8	1 slice	60
Melba Toast	.3	1 slice	16
Multigrain	2.0	1 slice	100
Pita	3.0	1 pita	210
Sourdough	.8	1 slice	90
Tortilla	1.0	1 large	150
Rye	1.0	1 slice	70
White Wheat	.8	1 slice	70
Whole Grain	2.0	1 slice	70
Buns	.8	1 bun	110
Pasta			
Noodles	2.7	1 cup	213
Spaghetti (enriched, cooked)	2.1	1 cup	197
Whole Wheat	6.6	1 cup	180
Nuts & Seeds			
Almonds	4.3	1 cup	910
Cashews (Roasted)	1.0	1 oz	170
Flaxseed, Linseed	4.8	1 oz	141
Macadamia	3.0	12 nuts	200
Mixed (Roasted)	2.0	20 nuts	200
Peanuts (Roasted)	2.0	35 nuts	166
Pecans (Roasted)	2.2	1 oz	195

Water:
How 8 Glasses a Day Keep Fat Away

As busy as the day gets, we usually forget about the importance of one other very important aspect of diet—water. If you remember your grade school science, you will remember that water is the universal solvent. That means that a whole bunch of chemical reactions can and do take place in the medium of water. From 40% to 60% of your body weight is water! Before anyone gets the crazy idea that you can lose a whole lot of weight if you deprive yourself from water, consider the following: dehydration places a great burden on the circulatory functions and severely impairs the body's capacity for thermoregulation. Heat is absorbed by water with only slight changes in temperature. What this means is that when you exercise and create excess heat, water helps to keep your body temperature stable. As soon as the body's core temperature rises too high, it will try to stop the source of heat production.

Also consider the fact that 72% of the weight of muscle is water and a mere 20 to 25% of fat's weight is water. So if you become dehydrated or lose a lot of water through improper "dieting," most of the water you will lose will come from your muscles! So the muscles will effectively shrink and function inefficiently while your fat hardly suffers a dent. With your muscles in a dehydrated state, they cannot perform their fat burning function very well at all. So that fat lives on happily ever after and your hard earned muscle literally shrinks away.

As incredible as it may seem, water may quite possibly be the single most important catalyst in losing weight and keeping it off. Although most of us take it for granted, water may be the only true "magic potion" for weight loss and permanent control.

***WATER SUPPRESSES THE APPETITE NATURALLY AND HELPS THE BODY METABOLIZE STORED FAT. Studies have shown that a decrease in water intake will cause fat deposits to increase, while an increase in water intake can actually reduce fat deposits. Here's why: The kidneys can't function properly without enough water. When they don't work to capacity, some of their load is dumped onto the liver. One of the liver's primary functions is to metabolize stored fat into usable energy for the body. But if the liver has to do some of the kidney's work, it can't operate at full throttle. As a result, it metabolizes less fat, and more fat remains stored in the body and weight loss stops.

***DRINKING WATER IS THE BEST TREATMENT FOR FLUID RETENTION. When the body gets less water, it perceives this as a threat to survival and begins to hold on to every drop. Water is stored in tissues and may show up as swollen feet, legs, and hands. Diuretics offer a temporary solution at best. They force out stored water along with some essential nutrients. Again, the body perceives a threat and will replace the lost water at the first opportunity. Thus, the condition quickly returns.

The best way to overcome the problem of water retention is to give your body what it needs—plenty of water. Only then will stored water be released. If you have a constant problem with water retention, excess salt may be to blame. The more salt you eat, the more water your system retains to dilute it.

***THE OVERWEIGHT PERSON NEEDS MORE WATER THAN THE THIN ONE. Larger people have larger metabolic loads. Since we know that water is the key to fat metabolism, it follows that the overweight person needs more water.

***WATER HELPS TO MAINTAIN PROPER MUSCLE TONE by preventing dehydration and by enhancing muscle's natural ability to contract. It also helps to prevent the sagging skin that usually follows weight loss. Shrinking cells are buoyed by water, which plumps the skin and leaves it clear, healthy, and resilient.

***WATER HELPS RID THE BODY OF WASTE. During weight loss, the body has a lot more waste to get rid of-all that metabolized fat must be shed. Again, adequate water helps flush out the waste.

***WATER CAN HELP RELIEVE CONSTIPATION. When the body gets too little water, it siphons what it needs from internal sources. The colon is one primary source. Result?

Constipation. But, when a person drinks enough water, normal bowel function usually returns.

How much water is enough? On the average, a person should drink eight, 8-ounce glasses every day. That's about two quarts. However, the overweight person needs more. The amount you drink also should be increased if you exercise or if the weather is hot or dry. Drinking at least one-half a gallon per day is recommended.

Water should preferably be cold—it is absorbed into the system more quickly than warm water. And some evidence suggests that drinking cold water can actually help burn calories.

When the body gets the water it needs to function optimally, its fluids are perfectly balanced. When this happens, you have reached the "breakthrough point." What does this mean?

- Endocrine gland function improves.
- Fluid retention is alleviated as stored water is lost.
- More fat is used as fuel because the liver is better able to metabolize stored fat.
- Natural thirst returns.
- There is a loss of hunger almost overnight.

If you stop drinking enough water, your body fluids will be thrown out of balance again, and you may experience fluid retention, unexplained weight gain, and loss of thirst. To remedy the situation, you'll have to go back, drink a lot of water, and force another "breakthrough."

Other benefits of water may be: reduced risk of kidney stones, lubrication of joints, good skin tone, relief of headaches, and decreased premenstrual bloating.

MORE ABOUT WATER...

Bottled water is, quite frankly, the wave of the future. More and more Americans are concerned about their health, the environment, and how our environmental problems affect our health. One in six people drink water with excessive amounts of lead, a heavy metal that impairs children's IQ and attention span. Yet this is the water our children are growing up on!

There are several types of bottled water, depending upon the source of the water. Clear distinction should be made between the sparkling waters (which are generally used as an alternative to soft drinks or alcoholic beverages, or used as a refreshment beverage) and bottled drinking water, which is consumed as an alternative to tap water and used for cooking and mixing with coffee, powdered mixes, etc. There is a clear distinction between the two types of bottled water, where they are purchased, and the price of each. Approximately 75 percent of bottled water comes from protected springs or wells, while 25 percent is derived from the same source as public water supplies.

Bottled water is the most highly regulated supply of drinking water. Bottled drinking water, like tap water, must meet standards outlined in the Safe Drinking Water Act and any subsequent standards adopted by the Environmental Protection Agency.

Because bottled water is considered a "food" by U.S. Food and Drug Administration, it is required to meet established criteria for sanitation and quality control procedures. All bottled water, including mineral water, must be processed and packaged in accordance with the FDA's Good Manufacturing Practice regulations (GMP), as well as any other regulations prescribed by local governments or country of origin.

Unlike public supplies, bottled water cannot be granted exemptions or variances for failure to meet federal quality standards. In a number of states, bottled water must test for and meet stricter standards than the public water supplies.

Water truly is our most precious resource, but few consumers really understand what's in it for them. While water covers over two-thirds of the earth's surface, only 1% is available for our use. Of that percentage, how much is really good for us? Here's a brief look at the water that we drink:

Public Water Supplies

Much of our municipal water supplies contain chemicals or contaminants such as lead, chlorine, fluoride, nitrates, sodium, pesticides, and/or insecticides. These products can lead to a weakened immune system, and some are suspected carcinogens.

Drinking Water

Drinking water comes from wells or public water supplies and has undergone at least a minimum treatment. Some bottled waters are actually "drinking water," even though "spring" may be in the name and/or on the label. The International Bottled Water Association (IBWA) is currently pushing for more stringent FDA labeling regulations.

Mineral Water

Mineral water contains more total dissolved solids (TDS), most of which cannot be used by the human body. In layman's terms, total dissolved solids include sodium, sulfates, nitrates, metals, and dissolved rocks. Therefore, the lower the number of total dissolved solids, the healthier the water is for you.

Distilled Water

Distilled water is basically "dead." Everything has been removed including the taste. Distilled water is perfect for steam irons and batteries but has none of the elements that gives water its good taste.

Spring Water

Spring water bubbles up naturally from deep in the earth, avoiding contaminants and debris. Spring water is usually the best-tasting water available. Naturally filtered as it makes its way to the surface of the earth, spring water is then purified under guidelines set forth by the IBWA (in compliance with state and federal regulations).

Doctors still recommend eight, 8-ounce glasses of water a day—but make sure that you're drinking the cleanest water available, not just a glass of chemicals! Read the labels, and contact your local treatment plant for an analysis of your water. The difference will be perfectly clear.

The fact is, spring water is the purest water available. Of all the different types of water available, spring water is the purest and healthiest.

Sodium (Salt)—Don't Add It

The night after a meal of pizza or Chinese food leaves most people with tightness in their hands and a bloated feeling. If they happen to step on the scales, they may notice a 3 to 10 pound weight gain. Certainly, this weight couldn't be fat from just one meal. More than likely, the gain is due to water retention.

To explain this phenomenon, we need to understand the role of sodium and water and their effects in the body. One gallon of water weighs approximately 7 pounds, and sodium attracts water very easily in the body. So, if a large amount of sodium is ingested, a larger amount of water is retained. This explains the large gain in pounds according to the scales.

Understanding the sodium/water connection, we can now discuss how this concept may cause health problems. The most common health problem associated with elevated sodium intake is hypertension.

Explaining this process physiologically is quite complex, but a very simple explanation is as follows: sodium is ingested, absorbed into the blood, and then attracts water into the blood.

This in turn, causes an increase in blood volume which causes an increase in blood pressure. This also causes increased demands on the kidneys, which will have a negative effect on blood pressure.

It is somewhat unclear to researchers and health professionals, why not all people are sodium sensitive. Therefore, not everyone will experience the harmful effects of sodium.

Typically, foods high in sodium are processed foods or fast foods like pizza, hamburgers, French fries, potato chips, Mexican food, Chinese foods, canned foods, and others that require large amounts of seasoning. Families who eat a lot of processed and convenience foods are consuming far more sodium than they need. Foods that are typically low in sodium are fresh or frozen fruits and vegetables, unprocessed meats, and the newer foods that are labeled "low sodium."

A simple guideline is that if a food contains more than 300 mg of sodium per serving, it should be avoided.

Most fast food establishments will provide a nutritional pamphlet that will give the breakdown of sodium per serving, as well as additional nutritional information. This is helpful when you are eating in restaurants.

Most people don't realize how pervasive sodium is in the American diet until they try to reduce their intake. You can exceed the body's minimum daily requirement of about 2000 milligrams without even trying. One cup of milk contains 120 milligrams. To help regulate sodium balance, water should be consumed liberally throughout the day—1/2 gallon at least. In closing it would be appropriate to say: "Don't add salt to food, since most foods contain sodium anyway." Eat healthy!

SODIUM CONTENT OF POPULAR CONDIMENTS, FATS, AND OILS

Product	Portion Size	Sodium (mg)
Salt	1 tsp	1938
Garlic salt	1 tsp	1850
Meat tenderizer (regular)	1 tsp	1750
Onion salt	1 tsp	1620
Soy sauce	1 tbsp	1029
Dill pickle	1 pickle	928
Baking soda	1 tsp	821
Teriyaki sauce	1 tbsp	690

Product	Portion Size	Sodium (mg)
MS6 (monosodium glutamate)	1 tsp	492
Baking powder	1 tsp	339
Green olives	4 olives	323
A-1 steak sauce	1 tbsp	275
French dressing (dry mix, prepared)	1 tbsp	253
Chili sauce (regular)	1 tbsp	227
French dressing (bottled, store bought)	1 tbsp	214
Worcestershire sauce	1 tbsp	206
Horseradish (prepared)	1 tbsp	198
Tartar sauce	1 tbsp	182
Italian dressing (dry mix, prepared)	1 tbsp	172
Catsup (regular)	1 tbsp	156
Thousand Island dressing (low calorie)	1 tbsp	153
Blue cheese dressing (low calorie)	1 tbsp	153
Margarine (regular)	1 tbsp	140
Russian dressing	1 tbsp	133
Barbecue sauce	1 tbsp	130
Pickle, sweet	1 pickle	128
Relish (sweet)	1 tbsp	124
Italian dressing (bottled, store bought)	1 tbsp	116
Butter (regular)	1 tbsp	116
Thousand Island Dressing (regular)	I tbsp	109
Pickles, bread and butter	2 slices	101
Mission olives, ripe	3 olives	96
French dressing (home recipe)	1 tbsp	92
Mayonnaise	1 tbsp	78
Butter (whipped)	1 tbsp	74
Mustard (prepared)	1 tsp	65
Chili powder	1 tsp	26
Tabasco sauce	1 tsp	24
Chili sauce (low sodium)	1 tbsp	11
Parsley, dried	1 tbsp	6
Catsup (low sodium)	1 tbsp	3

Product	Portion Size	Sodium (mg)
French dressing (low sodium)	1 tbsp	3
Butter (unsalted)	1 tbsp	2
Meat tenderizer (low-sodium)	1 tsp	1
Black pepper	1 tsp	1
Vinegar	½ cup	1
Margarine (unsalted)	1 tbsp	1
Oil vegetable (corn, olive, soybean)	1 tbsp	0

Grocery Shopping
"This is Where You Win or Lose!"

How to win the battle at the grocery store. Battle?? That's right. The way you win on your diet at home is first by winning at the grocery store. After all, if it is not in your cupboards or in your refrigerator, it is very hard to eat!

All that talk about willpower is hogwash! The only way to keep it out of your stomach is to keep it out of your home. If you've got a bag of chocolate chip cookies on the table, in a moment of weakness that whole thing is gone! You might as well forget about eating just one!

<u>Rule #1:</u> NEVER GO TO THE STORE HUNGRY.

You have probably heard this many times before, but it bears repeating. Also, if you take your family, don't let them go to the store hungry. Eat some fruit, or maybe several pieces, before heading off. This will help you stay rational when deciding what to buy. Hunger is a very strong drive. Being full will help clear your thinking process.

<u>Rule #2:</u> TAKE A LIST.

Determine what you need and stick to that list. Exclude frivolous junk foods. Fortunately, most cookies and candy are on the same aisle. Avoid that aisle altogether. Remember, once on the lips, forever on the hips. It is just not worth it to indulge in those chocolate covered, fat-laden, guilt-ridden treats. Get in the habit of being a good grocery shopper. It will save you money, too, since most of the forbidden foods are quite expensive.

Rule #3: BECOME A LABEL READER.

Make sure that you read the label to determine how much fat is in the product. If it is not listed in percentages or grams, then look at the list of ingredients. The ingredients are listed in order of quantity included in the product. If oil, margarine, whole eggs, or other fatty foods are listed at or near the top, BEWARE. This food is high in fat. By becoming a label reader you can keep your fat intake low and still eat lavishly.

PRODUCE: Get some fresh fruit and vegetables. Carrots are high in betacarotene. Celery requires as much energy to digest as it contains. Both of these have good nutrients and fiber. Tomatoes and lettuce are low in calories. Onions and bell peppers are great for preparing dishes.

LUNCHEON MEATS: Get the 98% fat free turkey slices or the lean chicken, avoid processed meats which are high in fat. Remember, the fat percentages advertised are misleading. Stick with the leanest of meats and count the grams.

CONDIMENTS: Get nonfat mayonnaise and dressings. Catsup and mustard are great. Some soy sauces are fat free, and add flavor to meat, but watch the sodium.

SEAFOOD AND MEAT COUNTER: Occasionally, oysters and shrimp are a real treat if not fried. Fish is an excellent source of low-fat protein, and is generally high in EPA oil, which has been shown to increase heart health. Turkey would be my next choice. Chicken, and occasionally ultra-lean ground beef is good. Even though lean ground beef may be advertised as 93% fat free, it is still higher in fat than turkey or chicken. Stick to the leanest of meat selections. Red meat eaten on a daily basis would make it impossible for you to keep your fat percentages in line. Depend more heavily on white meat.

SPECIALTY FOODS: The sauces of Mexican foods are all tomato-based and fat free. Avoid the fried taco shells and nachos. Italian food sauces are also tomato-based and very low in fat. Just make sure to read the label to see that no fat is added. Refried beans usually have fat or lard added, which is the worst kind of fat you could consume. Choose diet soups, and watch out for creamed soups.

CEREALS: Pick the cereals with the least amount of sugar and highest amount of fiber. Cheerios is a good cereal for kids. Children can become sugar addicts, which may cause them to be adult sugar addicts. Find adequate replacements for sugar-ladened cereals. Cereals with oat bran are good choices. Coco-Puffs are low in fat and may help wean you from your chocolate craving without loading on the fat.

CANNED VEGETABLES: Just make sure they are not packed with any type of oil.

SPICES: Spices, onions, and peppers are generally fat-free. Your diet doesn't have to be bland. With a little preparation, you can discover great tasting foods that help you keep the fat off.

CANNED MEATS: Tuna fish is an excellent source of protein. Make sure that it is packed in water. Mix tuna with the new non-fat mayonnaise, and you have a great tasting, healthy meal.

DAIRY: Skim milk is great for calcium and protein. Avoid 1% or 2% or whole milk. Children two and under, however, need whole milk. But, as they grow, if they tend to be overweight, switch to skim milk for them as well. Strolling down the dairy aisle, many people are stumped when they come to butter and margarine. Believe it or not, you can live without them. Even though they say "low-cholesterol," they are still pure fat! Learn to cook without it. A squirt of non-stick spray will do the trick. Get all the eggs you want, but separate the yolks and throw them away. Egg whites are the best source of protein for human consumption. They have the finest amino-acid balance. Nonfat yogurt is also tasty.

SNACKS: Fat free pretzels and fat free crackers are good, as well as low-fat, diet popcorn. Try rice cakes, too.

BREADS: Read the label and you can find a variety of non fat breads. Some pitas are nonfat. Bagels—especially the raisin-cinnamon kind—are a low-fat, tasty treat. Watch out for the caloric content!

DESSERTS: Popsicles that are sugar-free are good. There are numerous low-fat or nonfat frozen desserts to try. Also try diet puddings and fat-free cookies. Some pastries are now fat-free. *BEWARE: SUGAR THAT IS NOT USED BY THE BODY QUICKLY AS ENERGY IS CONVERTED INTO FAT!* Don't overload in this area, or you will gain weight and fat. Fruits with a dab of diet whipped cream are another healthy treat.

Other grocery shopping tips: Pre-basted turkeys are injected with saturated oils and may be high in salt and sugar. Also, do yourself a favor and don't wander through the inside sections of your store. You'll find most of a dieter's enemies along those aisles. By contrast, the outside aisles are much more "diet-friendly." Just think about it: in those outside aisles you find fresh fruits, vegetables, chicken, fish and dairy products.

As you win the battle in the grocery store, then you ultimately win the battle at home. In summary, know the nutrients of all the foods. You can do this simply by reading the label. Watch out for two things: the amount of fat content and the amount of sugar content. Keep these to a minimum. You will find that you can eat well, be full, and get leaner and healthier, all at the same time.

Eating Out

Rule #1: Plan, Plan, Plan

Decide ahead of time what you will eat when you get there. Decide about everything you will eat! Don't leave anything to chance or spur of the moment.

Rule #2: Ask, Ask, Ask

Inquire! Don't be afraid to ask a waiter or host how something is prepared. Watch out for little things hidden in the sauces and marinades.

Rule #3: Control, Control, Control

Exercise portion control. Serve yourself only what you know you should eat. Most restaurants serve portions much larger than you should eat. The concept of "I'm paying for it, so I might as well eat it" doesn't fit in too well with a low-calorie nutritional program.

Ten years ago, when I wrote my second version of "Shape Up," eating out was a real challenge to my low-fat, healthy diet. However, since then, restaurants have become savvy to the fact that consumers are health conscious.

Almost all of the fast-food chains are introducing low-fat meals. However, some still add needless fat-based dressings, which could be omitted to provide a healthy, low-fat dish.

You can limit fat and calories while eating fast foods. Basically, avoid beef, mayonnaise, fried foods, and fat-based sauces. Stick with grilled or broiled chicken, and ask that no butter be added to the meat or bread. Also, omit the cheese, which is extremely high in fat.

At Mexican fast-food places, don't eat the fried taco shells or nachos. Chicken fajitas are good without cheese.

At the salad bars, stay away from the potato salad, the pasta salad, and coleslaw—as well as any other salad that contain mayonnaise. Use "light" dressing or olive oil and vinegar instead of regular dressing.

At the potato bar, don't add butter or cheese. Catsup is the best choice for topping.

You may want to assemble your own "survival kit" to take along with you. Include nonfat dressing. When dining out in restaurants, here is a sample of items that may be included in your low-fat meals:

BREAKFAST:
> Scrambled egg whites (avoid yolks) Prepared without oil or butter
> Pancakes with fruit topping or limited syrup (no butter added)

Whole grain cereals
Whole toast with jelly (no butter)
Skim milk
Coffee
Fresh fruit/fruit juice
LUNCH:
    Chicken, fish, turkey (broiled, baked, or grilled)
    Baked potato (no butter)
    Salad (low-cal dressing)
    Vegetables (Prepared without fat)
    Turkey sandwich on whole wheat (no mayonnaise)
    Grilled or broiled chicken sandwich (no Mayonnaise)
    Fruit
SUPPER:
    Same as lunch

Avoid casseroles. Hors d'oeuvres of shrimp or oysters are better than nachos and cheese. Avoid fried hors d'oeuvres or those baked with oil and butter, as well as those served with lots of cheese. Feel free to specify when ordering what type of sauce you prefer and what you must avoid. Once you get tuned into what foods contain fat, it can become an easy habit to look at a menu and choose a healthy meal. Often I take a copy of this book with me to use the nutritional guide as reference. When you stay away from fat, you can eat more, get fewer calories, and continue on your maintenance or weight loss program. Don't be afraid to be assertive about your order. You may get some double takes or strange looks, but that's O.K. It is always amusing when the cook comes out to see the "fool" who just ordered a dozen scrambled egg whites (me!). It's your waistline, so be friendly.

Healthy Cooking: Tips and Recipes

Cooking Tips
- Never season vegetables with oil, meat, margarine or butter. If you want a butter flavor, use Butter Buds or

some type of substitute, but don't tamper with the integrity of the food itself by adding unnecessary fat.

- Stir-frying is good, but use non-stick spray.
- Never deep fry.
- If you must use oil, use olive oil which is high in Omega III fatty acids and is excellent for your heart by raising the good kind of cholesterol (HDL).
- Change traditional, high-fat meals into low-fat meals. Example, a traditional hamburger calls for:

  4 oz. beef

  Bun

  1 oz. cheese

  1 Tbsp. mayonnaise

  Mustard, lettuce, tomato, onion

  Change it to:

  4 oz. extra-lean ground beef

  Bun

  Nonfat cheese

  Nonfat mayonnaise

  Mustard, lettuce, tomato, onion

  By doing this, you save 274 calories and 32 grams of fat!!!
- Mexican dishes prepared with lean ground turkey or ultra-lean ground beef are low in fat and high in protein. Use nonfat cheese. Stay away from refried beans and fried chips, though. The sauces in Mexican dishes are tomato-based and low in fat.

Recipes
High Protein "Wonder" Muffins
1 cup powdered diet shake

1 cup powdered milk

1³/₄ cup egg protein

3 Tbsp. oat bran

1¹/₄ cup all purpose flour

1 Tbsp. baking powder

1 tsp. cinnamon

$^1/_4$ tsp. salt

Combine in mixing bowl.

In separate bowl, stir together:

8 egg whites

1 Tbsp. vanilla

1 cup honey

2 cups Kellogg's All-Bran cereal

$^1/_2$ cup water

1 cup applesauce or 5 pureed ripe bananas

(You may sprinkle cinnamon and sugar on applesauce muffins; also, you may sprinkle dropped nuts on banana muffins.)

Spray muffin pan with Pam. Fill full with batter. Bake in preheated oven (350 degrees to 375 degrees) for 10-12 minutes, or until toothpick inserted in center of muffin comes out clean.

Low-Fat Lasagna

$^1/_2$ box Lasagna noodles

Lean ground turkey, or ultra-lean beef Spaghetti sauce

Nonfat cottage cheese

Nonfat cheese

Cook lasagna noodles as directed on box. Drain. Brown meat; drain, and add enough spaghetti sauce to flavor. Layer in casserole dish: sauce/noodles/meat/noodles/ cottage cheese/noodles/meat/noodles/sauce and top with cheese. (You may layer as you prefer.) Cook in 350-degree oven for 30 minutes.

No-Fat Honey Mustard Salad Dressing

Combine

$^1/_2$ cup water

$^1/_4$ cup lemon juice

2 Tablespoons honey

1 Tablespoon prepared mustard
$1/2$ teaspoon paprika
1 crushed garlic clove
    Shake, chill.
    14 calories per tablespoon and no fat!

Pita Protein Treat

$1/2$ pita
3 packets Equal
$1/2$ cup nonfat cottage cheese
Cinnamon to taste
    Combine Equal, cinnamon, cottage cheese. Fill pita. Enjoy!

Chocolate Chip Protein Bars

$2^1/_4$ cup all purpose flour
1 tsp. baking soda
1 tsp. salt
$1/_4$ cup sugar
$3/_4$ cup firmly packed brown sugar
1 tsp. butter flavoring
6 egg whites
12 oz. package semisweet chocolate chips
1 cup chopped nuts
    Preheat oven to 375 degrees. In small bowl, combine flour, baking ,soda and salt; set aside. In large mixing bowl combine sugar, brown, sugar, butter flavoring and egg whites. Blend well. Gradually add in flour mixture. Stir in chocolate chips and nuts. (Mixture consistency will not be thick as regular cookie dough.) Spread mixture into cookie sheet pan. Bake for 10- 12 minutes.

Pizza

Low, fat, whole-wheat sub-sandwich bread
Pizza Quick sauce or spaghetti sauce
Lean ground turkey or Ultra-lean ground beef

Fat Free cheese

Brown and drain meat. Cut sub-sandwich bread in half and place in oven set on "Broil" until lightly toasted. Remove from oven.

Add sauce; add meat and cheese. Broil in oven until cheese is melted.

Other Tips About Fat

***2% and 1% milk are almost as fatty as whole milk. To really cut the fat, use skim milk.

***Leave off the salad dressing and croutons from your salad. Crackers are high in fat!

***Other low-fat or nonfat snacks: Pickles, dried fruit, diet popsicles, bagels, diet popcorn, Cracker jacks, diet drinks.

Low-fat substitutes:
• Use nonfat mayonnaise or mustard or catsup, instead of regular mayonnaise.
• Use low-fat popcorn or non-fat pretzels, instead of nuts or chips.
• Use egg whites in recipes, instead of whole eggs.
• Use nonfat salad dressing, instead of regular dressing.
• Eat whole-wheat toast, instead of bran muffins that are loaded in fat.
• Eat nonfat frozen yogurt, instead of ice cream.
• Use only low sugar jelly on your toast, instead of adding butter or margarine.
• Eat nonfat cereals, instead of high-fat granola-type cereals.
• Use non-stick sprays to prepare pans for baking, instead of coating with oils or butters.

Remember, fat is fat, as far as calories are concerned. Granted some fats are healthier than others are, but when it comes to losing fat from your body, 1 gram of fat is still 1 gram of fat. Don't be fooled by labels that say "cholesterol free" or "low fat." Read the label and see how many grams of fat per serving. Percentages may seem low, such as 2% milk, but 2% milk actually gets most of its calories from fat and contains 5 grams per 8 ounces. Margarine has as much fat as butter. Get used to cooking without any type of fat, margarine, oil, butter, etc. You will save a tremendous amount of unnecessary calories.

Chapter Four

EXERCISE—FEEL BETTER!

Why Is Exercise Necessary?

EXERCISE KEEPS YOUR METABOLISM RATE UP

Why is exercise necessary at all if you just want to get rid of unwanted pounds, Obviously, if you just starved yourself, you could lose weight. Starvation prison camps of World War II proved that. But the biggest mistake a dieter can make is starving himself—because the body perceives a threat, holds onto what fat it has, and slows down its metabolism (the rate at which the body uses food for energy). This is called the "starvation syndrome." The body fights to maintain its present weight, and the end result is that the body needs fewer calories to stay at the same weight.

Drastically cutting back on calories slows your metabolism down. The most successful way by far to counteract this starvation syndrome is by stimulating your metabolism through exercise. I advocate at least 15-20 minutes of some form of exercise every 12 hours. This will keep metabolism high and allow your body to burn more calories even while at rest.

People who lose weight by dieting alone will find that, when they reach their goal, their metabolism has slowed down so drastically that it seems indulging in even a carrot stick will cause them to gain weight! Sometimes they may gain back even more weight than they originally lost. This weight gain and weight loss is called the "yo yo" syndrome. This syndrome can be avoided by incorporating a new life style in eating and exercising.

Therefore, in order to properly shed fat, you need to (1) control your diet and (2) increase your exercise. If your objective is to gain a better shape as well, in addition to cardiovascular (aerobic) exercise, you will also need resistance (anaerobic) exercise.

Resistance exercise (weight training) will be discussed later.

EXERCISE BURNS ADDITIONAL CALORIES

One pound of fat is equal to 3500 calories. If you burn 500 calories or fat during an exercise session, and you exercise every day for 7 days, you will have burned off one pound (7 days x 500 calories = 3500 calories = 1 pound). You can see how you could lose weight simply by beginning an exercise program.

EXERCISE BURNS FAT

For a lifelong transformation of your metabolism, your body must become highly effective at eliminating unwanted fat—both during exercise and at rest. Fat is a slow-burning fuel. Sugar (glycogen, which is carbohydrates stored in the muscle) is a fast-burning fuel. A person can actually select the desired fuel by controlling exercise intensity. High effort exercise uses primarily sugar for fuel. Minimal effort exercise uses a larger proportion of fat for fuel.

Higher level exercise keeps your heart rate at 70% to 85% of its maximum rate. At this rate, your body burns mostly sugar for the first 30 minutes. Also, this exercising leaves you hungry soon afterwards because you just spent 30 minutes lowering your blood sugar level. (A drop in blood sugar is one of the mechanisms behind appetite.)

Minimal-intensity exercise keeps your heart rate at 60% to 70% of your maximum heart rate. The net effect of this type of exercise will be a dramatic increase in fat-burning potential. This occurs because during the first minutes of any exercise, when you keep you heart rate at about 65%, you begin to gradually convert stored fat into energy. At the end of one hour, you are using 99% body fat for fuel. So, the longer you exercise at the minimal intensity level, the more fat you burn.

To ensure exercise is in the best fat-burning range, use this formula:

220 minus your age = maximum heart rate

Maximum heart rate x .60 = 60%

Maximum heart rate x .70 = 70%

As an example, a 40-year-old, during exercise, should keep his heart rate between 108 and 126 beats per minutes

(220 - 40 = 180; 180 x .60 = 108 or 180 x .70 = 126)

Brisk walking (4 mph) is an ideal way to exercise in the minimal intensity range. Ideally, for optimal fat loss, you should exercise early in the morning for 15 minutes (minimum), which will stimulate your metabolism for the rest of the day. Take a longer walk in the evening.

Even though running for an hour would burn more calories than walking, your body cannot convert its own fat to energy at that fast pace, whereas walking at 4 mph. allows your body to efficiently use up (catabolize) its own fat stores of energy.

Your body tends to have its own set-point of weight and fat percentage, which is largely predetermined genetically. However, long aerobic exercise can actually fool your body into accepting a lower body-fat percentage. By the way, HDL, (the good cholesterol) is raised more significantly through regular long walks (2-1/2 to 5 miles daily) than, any other exercise. This, along with some strength training in the morning, is the very best combination.

The Best Exercise to Reduce Your Waistline

You may be wondering what type of sit-up I am going to describe. However, sit-ups don't reduce the waistline. They tighten the tummy, but they won't do anything to make it smaller.

The best singular exercise that you can do to reduce your waistline is WALKING! Remember, those long, brisk walks in which you keep your heart rate at 65% of its maximum are the best way to slim down. Isn't it great to know that you can shape up best by walking!

Walking is just one form of aerobic exercise, and generally the most convenient. However, swimming, bicycling, and other forms of exercise are equally beneficial. Any form of sustained movement that keeps your heart rate at between 60% and 70% will work.

Aerobics—Move It to Lose It!

Most people are familiar with the idea that aerobic exercise involves getting your heart rate up and keeping it there for a while by doing activities such as jogging, walking, using a step machine, etc. But that's not all there is to it if you want to obtain optimum results! Too many people begin an aerobic exercise program and lose hope after a couple of weeks because they aren't seeing the progress they were led to believe they should be seeing. So, let's get a few definitions straight before we go on.

Aerobic exercise is defined not by a type of exercise (like running, stepping, etc.), but instead by the energy system your body is using to fuel the exercise. Your body uses three primary energy systems, one of which is the aerobic system. Aerobic literally means "with air."

Those of you who are already performing some kind of resistance training will perhaps be concerned about losing muscle if you do too much aerobic work. Those of you who are already doing aerobics might be concerned you'll be doing too little work to lose fat. Neither should be concerned. Modifications can and should be made on an individual basis, depending on the desired effects (goals) and the results you are attaining. I only offer some recommendations and guidelines here. Before offering any suggestions, here's a formula that you should know:

Maximum heart rate = 220 - age
(in beats per minute)

This is an estimation of your maximum heart rate. If you are 30 years old, your maximum heart rate will equal 190 beats per minute (220 minus 30). Keep that in mind in the sections to come.

As a general rule, you can improve **aerobic capacity** if the exercise you are performing is at a sufficient capacity to increase your heart rate to about 70% of its maximum.

To calculate your training zone (where your heart rate should approximately be during training), you should multiply your age predicted max heart rate times 70%, or 80%, or 90%, keeping your heart rate within the limits of the 70 to 90% zone.

For your convenience, I have provided a chart (see Figure 1) to estimate the range of where your heart rate should be during aerobic exercise for maximum aerobic benefit. The first number represents the number of beats per minute, the second (bold) number represents the number of beats per 6 seconds.

Age	60%	70%	80%	90%
20	120/12	140/14	160/16	180/18
25	117/12	136.5/14	156/16	175.5/18
30	114/11	133/13	152/15	171/17
35	111/11	129.5/13	148/15	166.5/17
40	108/11	126/13	144/14	162/16
45	105/11	122.5/13	140/14	157.5/16
50	102/10	119/12	136/14	153/15
55	99/10	115.5/12	132/13	148.5/15
60	96/10	112/11	128/13	144/14
65	93/9	108.5/11	124/12	139.5/14

Figure 1. Age estimated heart rates based on % of MHR

Measuring your heart rate

To find your heart rate, you can use one of the following methods to indirectly measure it via a pulse. In each case, the measuring hand will utilize two or three fingers (index plus middle, plus ring finger).

Radial pulse—with pulse hand palm face up, place your fingers on your wrist just below the crease in your wrist. Press down gently to feel the pulse.

Carotid pulse—gently place your fingers on one side of your windpipe just below the level of your jaw. Press inwards very gently to feel the pulse.

By the way, if the thought of running hurts your knees or joints, try a treadmill that inclines. Set it up to 4 miles per hour and gradually increase the incline. You'll get your heart rate as high as you want without the joint pounding!

Why Exercise Makes You Feel Good

Exercise stresses many systems in our bodies. However, stresses created by exercise are not necessarily detrimental, and if properly controlled they can be used to elevate one's sense of physical and mental well-being. Exercise can produce feelings of euphoria and diminish the sensation of pain.

Research in the last 10 years has uncovered a highly specific hormonal system in the central nervous system (brain and spinal cord) underlying these effects. The diminished sense of pain and euphoria associated with exercise are produced by a family of substances that are chemically very similar to morphine—the endorphins. The endorphins mimic the action of morphine by reacting with specific regions of the brain and spinal cord to produce euphoria. These effects are well known to long distance runners and have been collected under the term of "runners' high." Most weight lifters and wrestlers are very familiar with the decreased sensation of pain during a workout or competition.

The stress of exercise also activates other physiological

systems before and during exercise. The adrenal glands located on top of the kidneys respond to exercise or the anticipation of exercise by releasing adrenaline into the blood. The adrenaline slows digestive functions, causes an increase in heart rate, a dilation of blood vessels in muscles and organs, and induces a sense of readiness or alertness in the person that is exercising or about to exercise.

The combination of adrenaline and endorphins generate a very strong sense of positive well-being in the person exercising.

Other Benefits of Exercise

- Exercise helps control cholesterol levels.
- Physically inactive people are more than twice as likely to develop coronary heart disease than those who exercise regularly.
- Regular exercise is now linked to reduce back injuries also.
- Regular exercise enhances the quality of life, and as we age it helps maintain our independence.
- Schoolchildren who exercise enjoy better health, better grades, and higher self-esteem.
- Exercising regularly lowers your resting heart rate.

And remember, exercise does not have to hurt to work. Taking four or five long, brisk walks per week greatly benefits your health.

Other Exercise Tips

- Drink a lot of cool water before, during and after exercise.
- During exercise, take only 10 seconds to measure your pulse rate. Otherwise, you could get an inaccurate reading. Why? Your heart rate plummets only 20 seconds after you stop exercising.
- Why mix exercise with dieting? If you just reduce the amount of food you eat, you will lose weight—but a lot of

what you lose will be muscle tissue. To increase the amount of fat you lose, you need to exercise as well. Also, muscle tissue burns a lot of calories. By increasing your proportion of muscle-to-fat, you increase your body's need for calories, and burn more.

- Forget elevators and escalators—take the stairs, instead. It's been said for every step you climb, you gain an extra four seconds of life! Climbing stairs also tones your legs and burns calories.

- If you want to keep off the weight you've lost, you better start exercising! In one study, men who had spent a year losing weight were split into two groups. One group tried to keep thin by eating less; the other by exercising more. The men who exercised gained less than two pounds.

- A walking tip: when you walk for fitness, walk up inclines. Then, in addition to toning your legs and thighs you're also trimming down your stomach, hips, buttocks, shoulders and arms!

- To improve your mood and beat the blahs, just get a move on! Just 20 minutes or so of moderate exercise should be enough to create the opiate-like hormones that are ultimately responsible for the so called "runners' high."

- Regular exercise may eliminate the need for drug therapy to control mild hypertension or high blood pressure. (Always consult your physician first.)

- Start off your morning with exercise. That way, your metabolic rate is increased for the entire day.

- You can't get a healthy, trim body cash-and-carry at the local gym. You only get it on the installment plan—and part of the payment is in regular sweat!

CALORIES BURNED/MINUTE

ACTIVITY	Your Weight in Pounds						
	100	120	150	170	200	220	250
Bicycling, 5.5 mph	3.1	3.8	4.7	5.3	6.3	6.9	7.9
Bicycling, 10mph	5.4	6.5	8.1	9.2	10.8	11.9	13.6
Calisthenics	3.3	3.9	4.9	5.6	6.6	7.2	8.2
Golf	3.6	4.3	5.4	6.1	7.2	7.9	9.0
Handball	6.3	7.6	9.5	10.7	12.7	13.9	15.8
Jogging	6.1	7.3	9.1	10.4	12.2	13.4	15.3
Raquetball	6.3	7.6	9.5	10.7	12.7	13.9	15.8
Squash	6.8	8.1	10.2	11.5	13.6	14.9	17.0
Swimming, breaststroke	4.8	5.7	7.2	8.1	9.6	10.5	12.0
Swimming, crawl	5.8	6.9	8.7	9.8	11.6	12.7	14.5
Tennis	4.5	5.4	6.8	7.7	9.1	10.0	11.4
Volleyball, moderate	2.3	2.7	3.4	3.9	4.6	5.0	5.7
Walking, 3 mph	2.7	3.2	4.0	4.6	5.4	5.9	6.8
Walking, 4 mph	3.9	4.6	5.8	6.6	7.8	8.5	9.7

To calculate the approxmate number of calories you burn during a single exercise, find the figure in the table closest to your weight, and multiply it by the number of minutes of continuous activity.

EXERCISE ACTIVITIES	CALORIES CONVERSION FACTOR
1) Walking (Leisurely)	(.037)
2) Golfing	(.038)
3) Gardening	(.044)
4) Rowing	(.046)
5) Tennis	(.050)
6) Cycling	(.054)
7) Walking (On hills)	(.055)
8) Swimming (Leisurely)	(.058)
9) Jogging	(.062)
10) Skiing (Cross-Country)	(.065)
11) Aerobic Dancing	(.076)
12) Circuit Weight Training	(.085)

Example: Using the formula to figure the calories burned in 60 minutes of exercise.

Specific Calorie conversion Factor x Body Weight x Minutes of Exercise = Calories Burned

Activity—Tennis, Factor—(.050), Body Weight—200 lbs.
Then, (.050) x 200 lbs. = 10 Calories per minute
So, 10 Calories x 60 minutes = 600 calories

Therefore, 600 Calories would be burned by a 200 lb. individual playing tennis vigorously for an hour.

God's Wisdom on Health

When examining the Scriptures, one can see that the food primarily consumed in Bible times was a great deal different from today.

I assume there were not a lot of refined sugars in the Bible times. Honey, however, was mentioned frequently, which was the main source of sweetening. Wheat was eaten before it was refined, so it was whole wheat, which is very high in fiber.

Concerning meat, fish was most often eaten, which is the best source of protein—low in fat, and with EPA oils that are good for the heart. The fatted calf was eaten only on an occasional basis as part of a celebration, such as when the prodigal son returned home.

In regard to exercise, walking was the primary mode of travel. Walking is the best form of exercise today, to slim and trim, and to help your heart stay healthy and happy.

The Bible stresses moderation in all things, and condemns gluttony. Jesus Christ gave us the prime example in the way that he lived, walked, and ate while he was here. He fed the multitude with whole grain bread and fish.

The primary oil used was olive oil, which is the healthiest oil to use for cooking or dressing. It actually helps raise your HDL—the good kind of cholesterol.

Let's Make a Commitment

Having worked with more than 1,000 individuals on improving their health through diet and exercise, one common trait was shared by all who were successful in their quest. They made a commitment to make a positive life-style change. Each person decided that it was time for a change. They were tired of feeling overweight, of clothes not fitting properly, of being stressed, and sluggish. With these feelings as a strong motivation, it was easy for them to commit to a long-term life-style change.

The first step in commitment to change is education. This book will provide you with the information you need. Second, time must be set aside for the change. Specifically, there needs to be time spent on planning meals, and time set aside for exercise. Proper planning will help you make choices that are healthy ones. The last step to successful commitment is being consistent with your new life-style. If you blow your diet, get back on track the next meal, not the next day. If you miss a workout, make it up.

In most instances, the nutrition plan described in the chapter on healthy eating will be the bedrock of your shape-up plan. You should not really think of this as a diet, but rather the basis for your new healthy life-style. If you're overweight when you begin, you will lose weight at a reasonable rate and not be too troubled with hunger or deprivation. It's a sensible approach to weight loss and control that will become a pleasant part of your new way of life.

Chapter Five

WEIGHT TRAINING

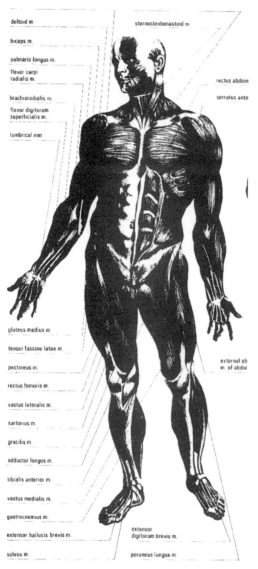

deltoid m.
biceps m.
palmaris longus m.
flexor carpi radialis m.
brachioradialis m.
flexor digitorum superficialis m.
lumbrical mm.
gluteus medius m
tensor fasciae latae m.
pectineus m.
rectus femoris m.
vastus lateralis m.
sartorius m.
gracilis m.
adductor longus m.
tibialis anterior m.
vastus medialis m.
gastrocnemius m.
extensor hallucis brevis m.
soleus m.
sternocleidomastoid m.
rectus abdom
serratus ante
external ob m. of abdo
extensor digitorum brevis m.
peroneus longus m.

This can help you understand which muscles do what. All muscles have a point of origin and insertion—variance in these points can give a leverage advantage or disadvantage. Muscles never push; they are only able to contract or pull. You can't increase the amount of muscle cells or fibers, but you can greatly enlarge the ones you have. By adding weight, your body tries to compensate for the added burden, and the muscles are stimulated to grow. Muscle operates on a use or lose principal. When the burden is no longer there the muscles begin to atrophy and shrink; however, they come back easier the second time than at first.

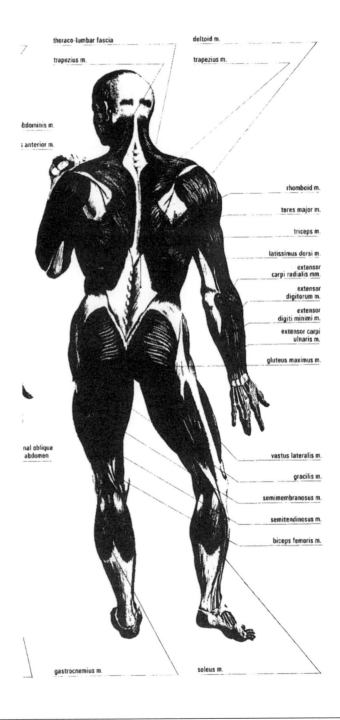

thoraco-lumbar fascia

trapezius m.

deltoid m.

trapezius m.

bdominis m.

s anterior m.

rhomboid m.

teres major m.

triceps m.

latissimus dorsi m.

extensor
carpi radialis mm.

extensor
digitorum m.

extensor
digiti minimi m.

extensor carpi
ulnaris m.

gluteus maximus m.

nal oblique
abdomen

vastus lateralis m.

gracilis m.

semimembranosus m.

semitendinosus m.

biceps femoris m.

gastrocnemius m.

soleus m.

Important Note

Don't be afraid to lift weights or train on machines. It may be one of the best new experiences you've ever had!

As you implement this part of your exercise program, your body will become a more efficient fuel burner. The more muscle you have, the more calories you use at rest or movement. You'll be able to eat more without getting fat, and do more without getting tired, and look more and more fit as each month goes by. So get started and stick with it—YOU'LL BE VERY GLAD YOU DID!

Body Building for All Ages

There is no age at which weight training is not beneficial. It can benefit the 9-year-old and the 90-year-old. It increases muscle strength, muscle size, muscle flexibility, as well as bone density. It is good for your heart, lowers blood pressure, and increases cardiovascular fitness. All of these benefits are available when done with a minimal degree of intensity and on a regular basis. It will not cause you to be muscle-bound, and will not restrict your range of motion. For most, weight training will not cause you to look like Arnold Schwarzenegger (unfortunately). It will not make women unattractive. As a matter of fact, almost all Miss America contestants lift weights.

The degree of lifting you should do depends on what you want to accomplish. There are three stages: beginning, intermediate, and advanced. You may always wish to keep this part of your exercise at a minimum. If so, you can stick with the beginner's routine. However, if you want to gain more shape and use of your body, you may want to increase to the intermediate or advanced. There is also a recommended program for high school athletes. This routine is for off-season, but it can be reduced and continued through the season as well.

Remember, you can make significant gains at any age. I've

been lifting 30 years, both as a competitor in bodybuilding and power lifting. I've competed with phenomenally well-built, strong men and women who started later in life and who are now well into their 60s—people who started to get in shape and then took competition up as a healthy hobby. This kind of exercise really makes you feel good and has wonderful rewards!

General Rules for Lifting

Any time you start a new program, start easy. Begin with just one set and increase one set per workout until you reach the full workout. This will reduce the potential for soreness. Also, taking aspirin with your pre-workout meal at the beginning of your workout will help prevent soreness and joint problems.

You have probably heard that you should not work out every day. It is, however, OK to lift every day, but only work each muscle group twice a week, giving plenty of time for recuperation. Remember, muscles grow between workouts so the resting is important. These workout plans let each muscle group rest at least two days between use.

Even if you want to get big and strong, 20 minutes of concentrated, intense work per muscle is plenty. A light protein and carbohydrate snack is very helpful 30-45 minutes after you work out. That's when the nutrient uptake is peak as the muscle begins to recover and grow. Three or four sets of three or four different exercises are plenty, even for the most advanced trainer.

Toning and firming can be accomplished with just two-four sets per muscle twice a week.

Sleep plays an important part in recovery. Make sure you get all you need, especially if you want to grow.

Remember, do each exercise with good form. Don't worry about how much weight you use. It's better to start light and do concentrated, smooth reps—don't use jerky movements. Then add weight as you progress.

Beginning Bodybuilding

This can be done either in a local health club or at home. Ladies can use a simple set of plastic dumbbells that weigh about 5 or 10 pounds each. Men can use a little heavier set of dumbbells. We are going to start from the top down.

While sitting, pick the dumbbells up off the floor, swing them up to your shoulders, and press them overhead. Do this for 10 repetitions, rest for one minute and do 10 more repetitions, then rest and do about 10 more, (three different sets). Next, lower your hands back down and do lateral raises, keeping arms extended and your elbows locked. Raise your arms up with your palms facing down until the dumbbells come up approximately to just above the top of your head and then back down. Do this also for three sets, 10 each set. Then lie on a bench on your back with the dumbbells, your arms slightly bent. Drop the elbows down and do bench presses, three sets of 10 reps each. Then "flys," with arms slightly bent and the weights from below your chest up over your chest where they touch and back down—three sets of 10. Then stand up and bend your back parallel to the ground and your knees slightly bent and slowly pull the dumbbells up to your chest all the way up and then back down for three sets of 10. Then with your legs locked and a dumbbell in each hand, do dead lifts where you start with the weight of the dumbbells on the floor keeping your knees locked and using your lower back to stand back up erect, and then back down again. Do three sets of 20. Then standing, do curls with your palms facing up. Curl the weight up to your shoulder keeping your arms close to your side for three sets of 10. Do this exercise routine on Mondays, Wednesdays, and Fridays.

Rest approximately one minute between each set of 10 repetitions.

Start off slowly with a weight that is comfortable and gradually increase as you get stronger and are able to handle the weights more easily. This workout won't build a great deal of muscle mass, but it will help shape your body and get those muscles toned, and improve bone density. This is a workout that can be done by anyone at any age.

Exercises for Different Body Parts

There are many different types of exercises you can do for each body part. You might even create some of your own. However, the following exercises are the main exercises that power lifters, body builders and weight lifters perform. The following are the body parts listed with the name of the primary muscle and secondary muscles worked in each exercise.

NECK

There are four basic neck movements—side to side and front to rear. This can best be done in a machine or with a partner pushing, while you resist pushing, on the side of the head until the ear touches the shoulder. Repeat from the other side. Also, push the head back and then pull it forward until the chin touches the chest.

CHEST

Bench press primarily works the pectoralis major and the pectoralis minor muscles. Secondarily, it works the frontal deltoids and triceps. This can also be done with dumbbells.

Incline bench press—done on a fairly steep angle on an incline bench. This works your upper pectorals primarily and your frontal deltoids. This is popular with girls in developing that center line cleavage in the upper chest. This also uses the frontal deltoids secondarily and triceps and can also be done with dumbbells.

SHOULDERS

Seated military press—behind the neck, works the entire deltoids. There are three parts to the deltoid: front, center, and rear. The military press behind the neck works the whole deltoid area. Secondarily it works the trapezius and triceps. This can also be done with the dumbbells.

Upright rows—also develop deltoids and trapezius.

Dumbbell flys—done laterally with palms down, work the whole deltoid area and is a great help in widening the deltoids.

Front deltoid raises—work the front part of the deltoid.

Bent-over deltoid raises or flys—work the rear deltoid, which is sometimes difficult to work. Other muscles worked in this are the trapezius.

TRAPEZIUS

The primary purpose of the trapezius muscle is to pull the shoulders up and back. These muscles are best worked by doing shoulder shrugs and power cleans.

ARMS

The arms are broken down into two basic parts:

Biceps—these are best worked by a variety of curls (both dumbbell and barbell). For building the highest peak and bulk on the biceps, I like straight bar standing curls with as heavy a load as possible without cheating, doing slow rhythmic motions. Doing curls with a special curl bar on a preacher bench or Scott bench helps to isolate the biceps. Seated dumbbell or hammer curls are also an excellent exercise for building shape and size.

Triceps—these are involved in every pushing and pressing movements, but to get optimum growth requires extra isolated work. I like three tricep exercises. 1) Lying on a bench with a fairly close grip on the bar—come down, with your upper arms perpendicular to the floor and with your elbows acting as a pivot, touch just below your forehead with the bar and straighten back up. 2) Close grip bench presses—done on a regular bench like regular bench presses except holding your hands close together. If you can do it without straining your wrists, you should let your thumbs touch each other when they stretch out. 3) Standing pull-downs-pull a pulley, keeping your elbows against your stomach and using only your triceps to force the bar down.

FOREARMS

Forearms are used in both tricep and bicep exercises as well as any time you squeeze your grip. Normally they don't need isolated work, but if you have a problem with forearm development, you could do wrist curls backwards or forwards. Sit on a bench, let your wrist hang over your knees keeping your wrist on top of your knees and curl the bar up and down with just your hand moving only a few inches with each motion. Reverse curls, standing doing a regular curl except reversing the grip is also good for building the top part of the forearm.

LATS—Latissimus Dorsi

Any pulling motion uses your lats. The two best exercises are sitting on a lat machine pulling the bar from above your head down behind your neck or in front of your neck. Do sets of 12 repetitions, as your lats respond better to higher repetitions. Alternate pulling the bar behind your neck and the next set in front of your neck. This works your lats from two different angles. The other helpful lat pull is sitting on the floor doing a rowing type motion on a cable machine, pulling the handle to your chest and then pushing it forward until your arms are fully extended again. If you don't have a machine-stand with the bar on the floor, bend over so your back is parallel with the ground. It is better to brace your head if you have lower back problems as this alleviates some of the stress. Pull the weight up to your chest and then back down.

ABDOMEN

There are two basic muscles to work in the stomach. One is the rectus abdominis, the muscle that runs from your groin to your chest. This is worked best by doing crunches or a variety of sit-ups. The other muscle, your external oblique, runs like a rubber band around your stomach, and is the muscle that is underneath the love handles, as they are called, where fat is often deposited. It can be worked by putting a dumbbell in one hand at a time and doing side bends.

LOWER BACK

This muscle is worked primarily in the dead lift doing slow rhythmic motions. Standing, with feet shoulder width apart, grasp the bar at shoulder width; stand erect till your hands are between your waist and your knees, and then back down. This develops overall body strength but primarily uses the lower back muscles. You may either do these stiff-legged with less weight or additional weight and bend your knees.

GLUTEUS MAXIMUS

This is the largest muscle in the body. This is your hip and it's worked best in the squat. The deeper you go, the more it is worked. You don't see real big buttocks on a lot of body builders like you do on powerlifters whose gluteus maximus muscles are more powerfully developed.

THIGHS

Quadriceps are developed primarily through regular squats, and to get additional growth and development for the tops of the quadriceps, do front squats and/or back squats. Regular squats are done by placing the bar on the shoulders behind the neck, spreading your feet about shoulder width, with your feet just slightly pointed out. Squat down until your thighs are parallel with the ground and then stand erect. Do front squats the same way except hold the bar in front of your neck (which is difficult to do until you are used to it). Set the bar on your shoulders and hold it there with your hands. Front squats force you to stay straight, placing more stress and building more muscle around the knee and the top of the thigh. Hack squats can be done on a machine or on the floor by doing a dead lift type exercise, except the bar is behind your ankles instead of in front and the heels are elevated. If, for some reason, you can't do front squats and you want to develop more muscle around the knee area, it will help to do regular squats with your heels placed on a 2" x 6" board.

HAMSTRINGS-BICEPS FEMORIS

This muscle is developed by doing stiff-legged dead lifts with your feet elevated on 4" of wood or by doing leg curls on a machine. Unless you are a competitive body builder, regular squats will give you good overall leg development.

CALF-GASTROCNEMIUS

To get the most effective growth, the calf muscle should be worked standing up with your knees locked, the weight placed on your shoulders, and your toes on a 4-inch elevation so that you can stretch all the way down and all the way up. Donkey calf raises (where your knees are locked and you are bent over at the waist with somebody sitting on your hips) is a very effective way to work your calves without special equipment. The other way to work your calves is seated on a calf machine. For best development do these standing and seated!

Description of Specific Exercises

LEG PRESS

Place your feet on the platform with heels about shoulder width apart. Toes should be pointed out slightly (about 20 to 30 degrees). At the lowered position, your knees should form a 90 degree angle. At the extended position your knees should be unlocked to maintain tension on the muscles being worked. Breathe out on the pressing motion, breathe in on the return (with legs bending) motion. Make sure your knees stay over your feet (do not allow your knees to wobble together or apart). When you press the weight up, press through your heels, actually lifting the ball of your foot off of the platform.

LEG EXTENSION

The pad should be slightly above ankle level. Breathe out on the extension, and breathe in on the return (legs bending). Extend your legs fully, and hold the top (contracted) position for two seconds. Slowly lower your legs to the 90 degree position, maintaining tension on the quadriceps. Keep your ankles in a neutral position. Do not point the toes out or in.

STIFF LEG DEAD LIFT

With the knees slightly bent, bend over from the waist, being sure not to arch your back fully (some slight arching is alright) and grab a barbell. By thrusting forward with your pelvis, allow the hands and arms to act as hooks while you lift the weight up using your hamstrings and buttocks. Keep lifting until you are standing erect (not leaning back). Slowly lower the bar down to the front of your shins, only going as low as your level of flexibility allows. Breathe out on the lift, and in on the lower.

LEG CURL

The pad should be slightly above ankle level. Breathe out on the curl, and breathe in on the return (legs straightening). Curl your legs fully, and hold the top (contracted) position for 1-2 seconds. When curling the weight up, curl as high as you can, but do not allow your hips to flex, or buttocks to rise up. Keep your ankles in a neutral position. Do not point toes out or in. At the bottom (straight legged) position, do not relax the legs—maintain tension on the hamstrings.

CALF PRESS (ON LEG PRESS)

Place the balls of your feet on the end of the platform, with knees just slightly unlocked. Press the platform such that your ankles are fully plantar flexed (feet pointed). Make sure you press as far as possible. Slowly lower the platform, allowing your ankles to flex. Breathe out on the pressing motion, breathe in on the return (ankles bending). Press through the balls of your feet, almost trying to come up onto your toes.

BENCH PRESS

Lie on the bench with feet up (either on the bench or on a stool) so that the back can be flat. Grab the bar so that the distance between your hands is that distance your hands are apart when your arms are at 90/90. Slightly roll your shoulders back, allowing your chest to stick upward. Unrack the barbell, and slowly lower the bar to your chest at nipple level. Do not rest the bar on your chest! Slowly press the bar back up to just before your elbows lock. Maintain constant tension on your chest. If necessary, use isometric pressure by pressing the hands together (though there will be no motion because you are securely holding the bar). Breathe out when the bar ascends (when you press the bar up), and breathe in when the bar descends. Do not allow your elbows to flare out to the sides too widely. The angle between your torso and your upper arm should be no more than 80 degrees.

LAT PULL DOWN

Hold the bar with an overhand grip so that your pinkies are over the break in the bar. Your thumbs should be in a false grip (over the bar, wrapped over in the same manner as your fingers). Feet should be flat on the floor, abdominals contracted. Lean back slightly to allow the bar to travel in front of the body. Without bending the elbows, pull the bar down so that your shoulders are lowered (set) down. This is the start and finish position. Pull the bar down slowly, allowing your elbows to travel to your sides. Imagine your hands are hooks, and that you are trying to touch your elbows together through your body. At the bottom of the motion, squeeze your shoulder blades down and back. Slowly allow the bar to return to the top position, maintaining tension on the lats. Breathe out when pulling down, breathe in when allowing the bar to return to the top position.

SHOULDER PRESS

Sit with feet flat on the floor, back supported. Hold the dumbbells at shoulder height, with elbows at sides, and hands pointed toward the ceiling. Keep stomach tight during the exercise. Press up, moving only through the middle three fifths of the range of motion. Breathe out on the press up, in on the return.

TRICEPS PRESS DOWN

Using a rope attachment, stand with your knees slightly bent and your stomach held tight. Hold the rope, and bring your elbows to your sides. They will stay at your sides during the entire set. Slowly press your arms down, keeping your wrists locked, and flaring your hands/lower arms out to the sides. Extend your arms fully, and hold the contraction for 1 - 2 seconds. Slowly allow your arms to return to the top position, keeping elbows at sides. Do not relax at the top of the motion—maintain tension on the triceps! Breathe out on the press down, breathe in on the return to the top position.

BICEPS CURL

Using dumbbells, keep palms turned up, with wrists slightly bent back. Stand with elbows at sides, slightly anterior to midline to keep tension on the biceps. Keep knees slightly bent and stomach held tight. Slowly curl the weight up, keeping wrists bent back. Contract tightly at the top position. Slowly lower the weights to just before full extension, keeping tension on the biceps. Breathe out on the curl, in on the return to extension.

CRUNCHES

Lie on your back, with your legs up on a chair so that your hips and knees are bent to approximately 90 degrees. Keep your legs relaxed. Clasp your hands behind your neck, and flare your elbows out to the sides. Relax your head in your hands. Press your back into the floor, and raise your head and shoulders off of the floor as your stomach contracts slightly. This is your beginning and ending position. From here, slowly crunch up, and then lower down, maintaining tension in your abdominal muscles. Make sure you are not jerking upward!

All of the following photographs illustrating previously described exercises were taken in Tom's American Fitness Center using staff, personal trainers and members to demonstrate.

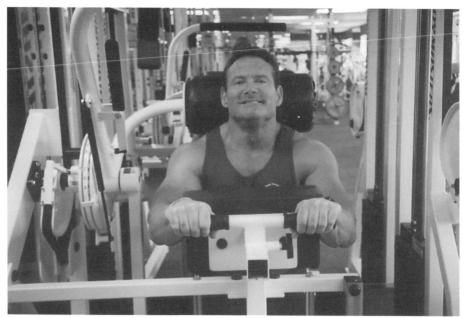

Back of Neck

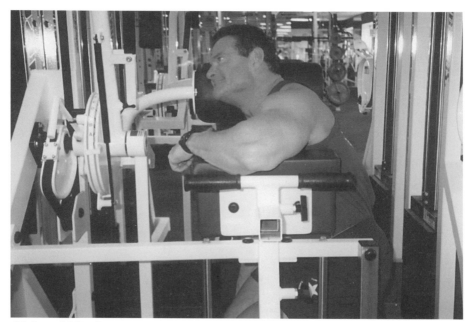

Side of Neck

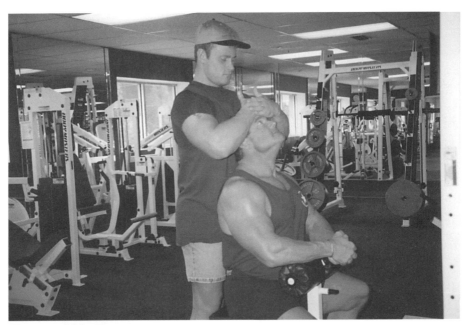

Front of Neck

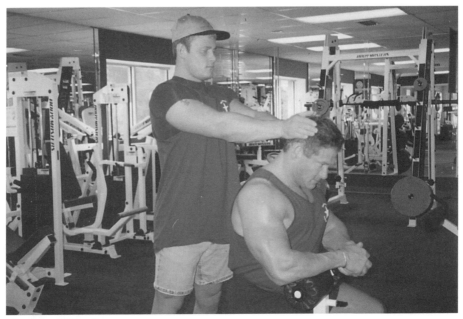

Back of Neck

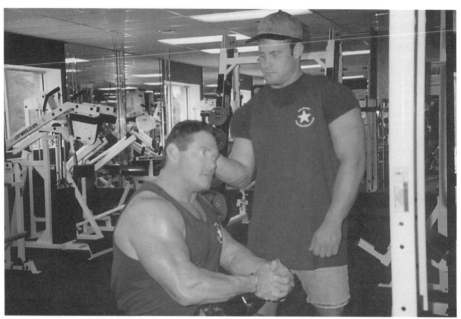

Side to Side—Neck

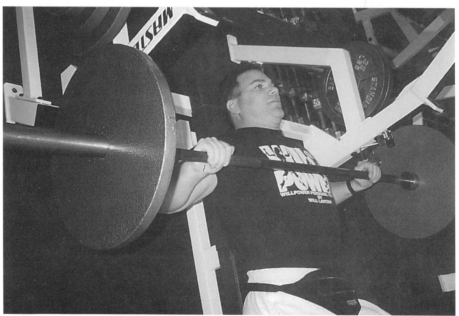

Chest—Barbell Bench Press

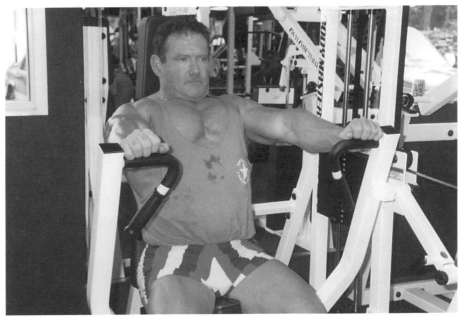

Chest—Machine Bench Press

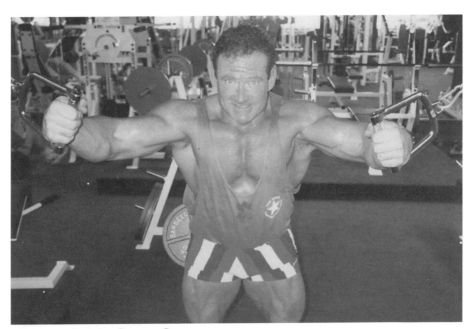

Chest—Cable Cross Over

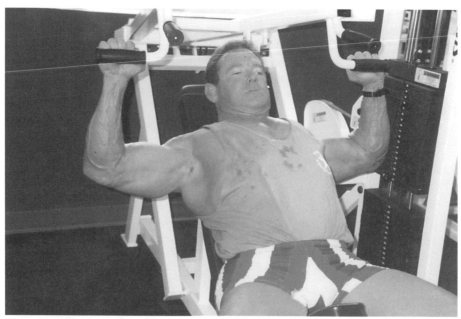

Upper Chest—Machine Incline Bench Press

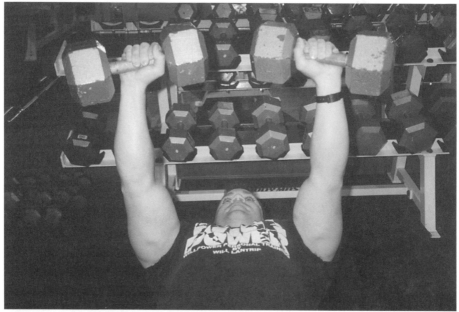

Chest—Dumbell Bench Press

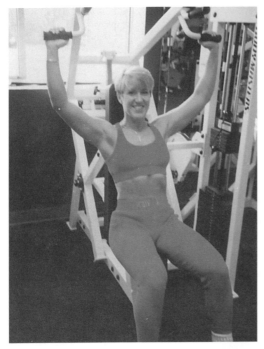

**Shoulders—
Machine Press**

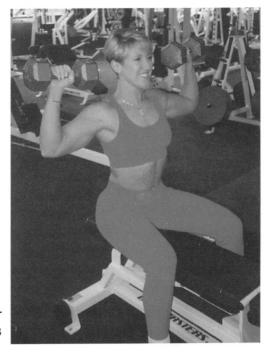

**Shoulders (Deltoids)—
Dumbell Presses**

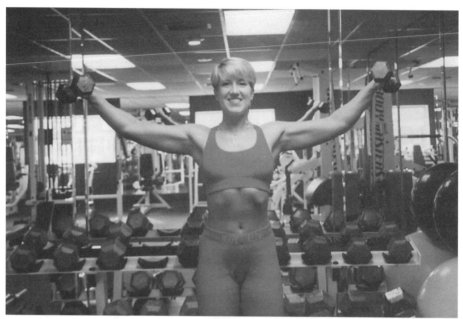

Dumbell Shoulder Lateral Raise

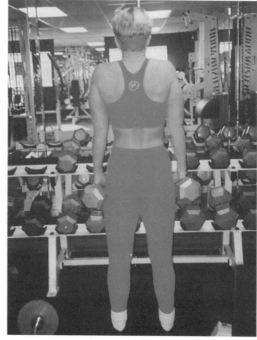

**Trapezius
Shoulder Shrugs**

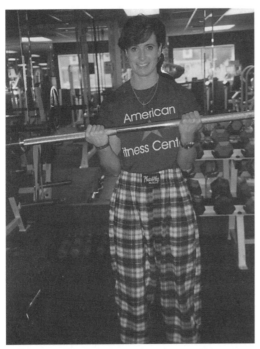

**Biceps—
Straight Bar Curls**

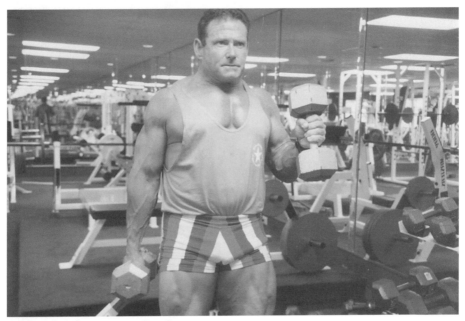

Biceps—Hammer Curls

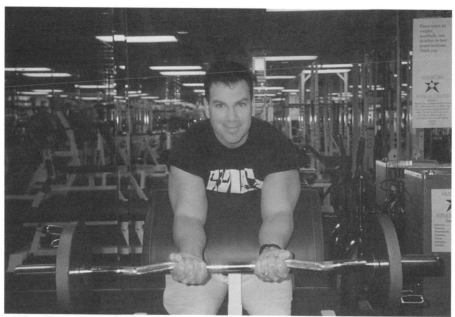

Biceps—Preacher Bench Curls

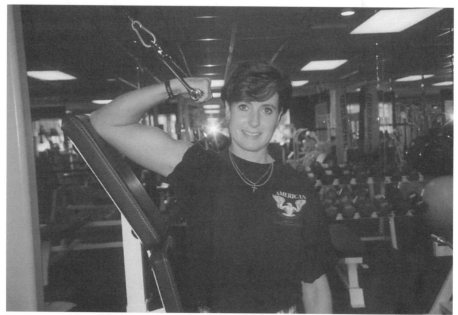

Biceps—Cable Concentration Curls

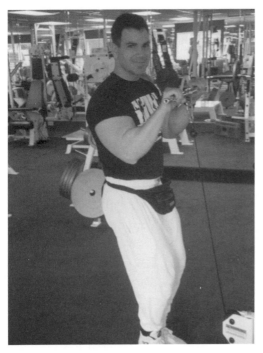

**Biceps and Forearms—
Reverse Cable Curls**

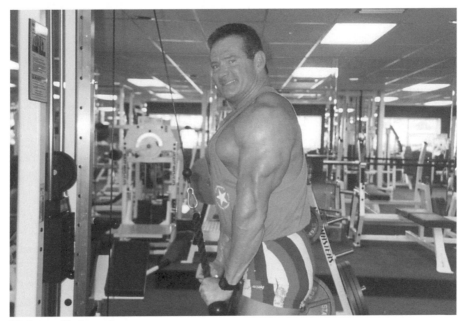

Tricep Extension

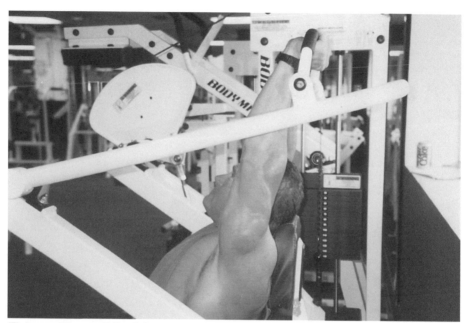

Tricep Press Machine

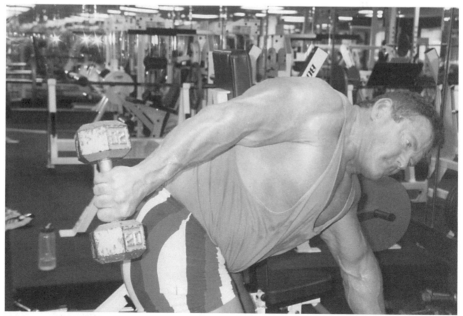

Tricep Kickbacks

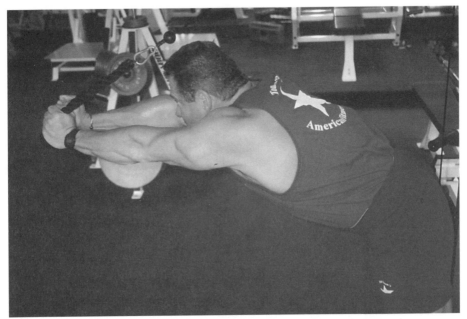

Triceps—Cable Extension

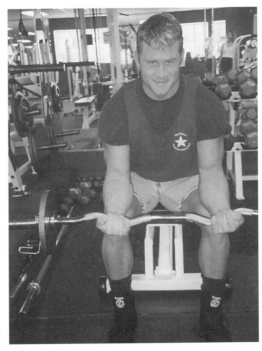

Forearms—Wrist Curls

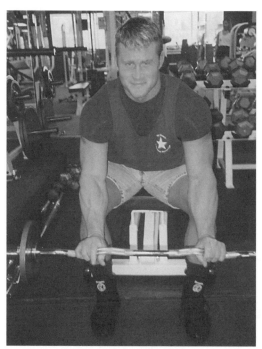

Top of Forearm—
Reverse Wrist Curls

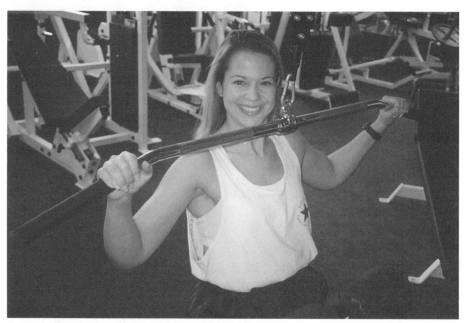

Lats—Pull Down to Top of Chest

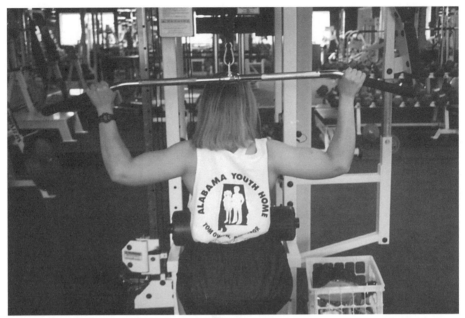

Lats—Pull Down Behind Neck

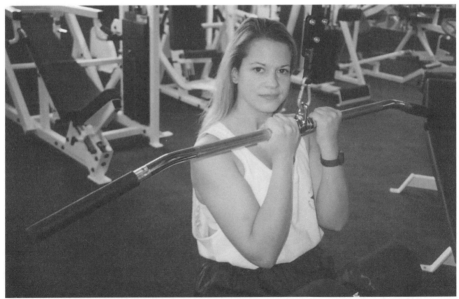

Lats and Upper Center Back Rhomboidei—Close Grip Pull Downs

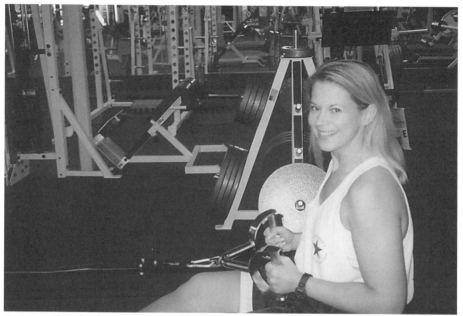

Lats—Seated Rows

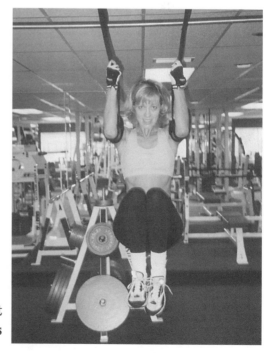

**Abs—Hanging Front
Leg Raises**

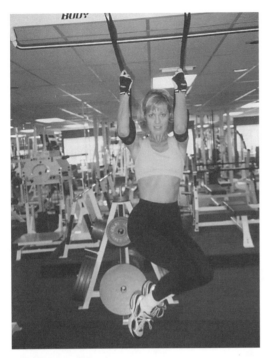

Abs—Hanging Leg Raises To The Side

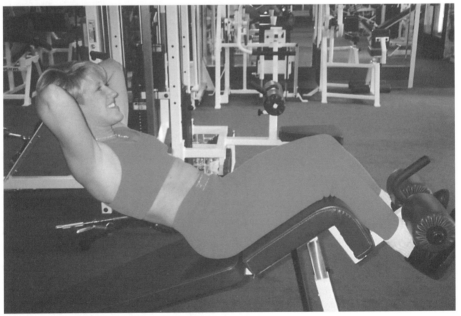

Abdominals—Incline Situps

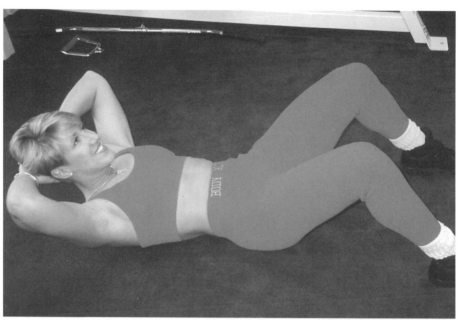

Abs—Crunches

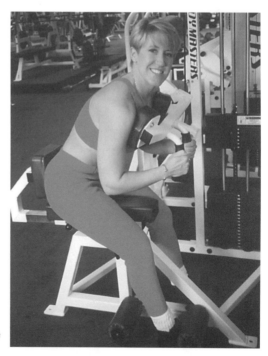

Ab Machine

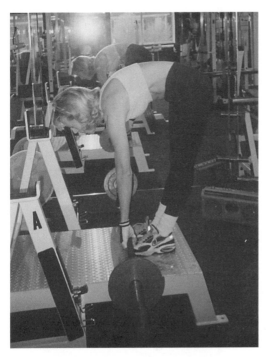

Low Back and
Hamstrings—Stiff
Legged Dead Lift

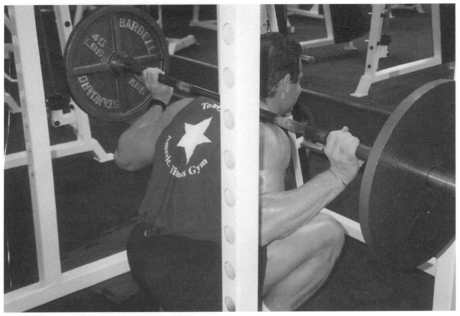

Thighs and Hips—Full, Deep Squats

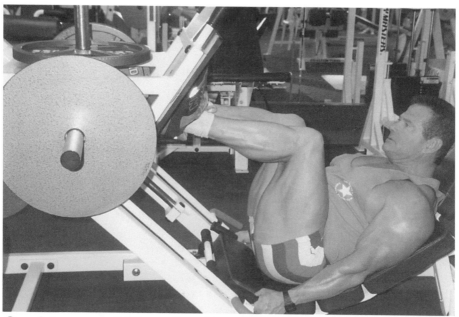

Quadriceps and Hips—Leg Press Machine

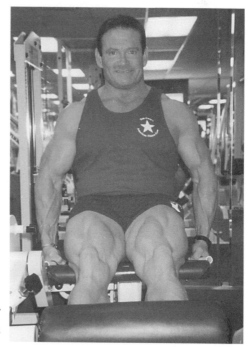

**Quadriceps—
Thigh Extension**

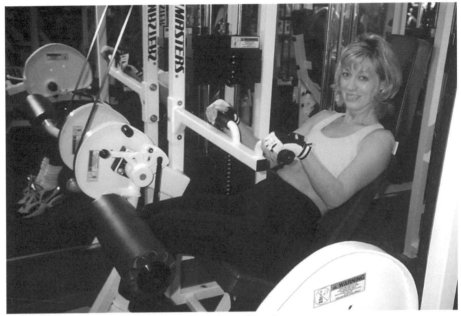

Hamstrings—Seated Hamstring Curl

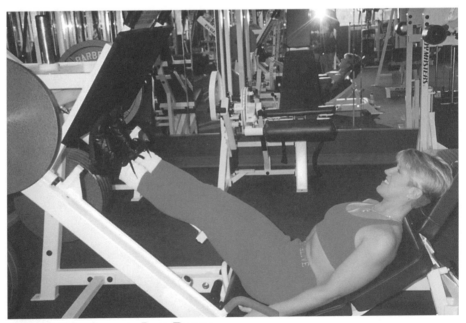

Calf Extension on Leg Press

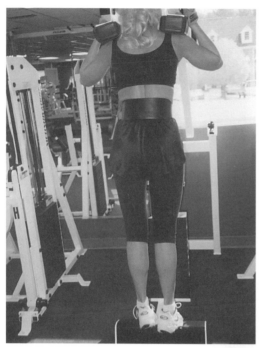

Standing Calves

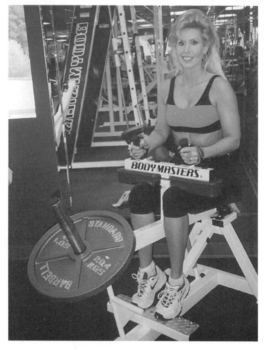

Seated Calves

The 10-10-10 Workout (intermediate)

This is good for men and women of all ages who are just beginning a workout program.

Day 1: 10 minutes on quadriceps (Squats 4 x 10)
10 minutes on hamstrings (Leg curls 3 x 10)
10 minutes on calves (4 x 25—Calf stretch in between)

Day 2: 10 minutes on chest (Bench press 2 x 10; Incline bench press 2x 10; and Dumbbell flys 2 x 20)
10 minutes on shoulders (Military press 2 x 10; Upright rows 2 x 10; and Standing flys 2 x 10)
10 minutes on triceps (Extension 2 x 10; Pulldowns 2 x 10)

Day 3: 10 minutes on lats (Pulldowns 2 x 10; Lat rows 2 x 10) 10 minutes on biceps (Curls 2 x 10; Standing barbell 2 x 10; and Seated dumbbell curls 2 x 25) 10 minutes on abdominals (Crunches 2 sets to failure; and Leg ups 2 sets to failure).

Day 4, 5, and 6 same as 1, 2, and 3. Take Day 7 off completely.

This is a good workout for toning, firming, and strengthening. It will not cause you to gain bulk, but it will give you a much better shape for a bare minimum workout. You could cut this in half and make it a 5-5-5 (or 15 minutes per day, 6 days per week) for a good beginner routine.

20-20-20 Workout

This is the exercise program that I recommend the most for people who are serious about reshaping their bodies and staying in shape. The 20-20-20 simply stands for 20 minutes on one body part, 20 minutes on another body part, and then 20 minutes of aerobic exercise. This is done six days a week for optimum effectiveness.

On Day 1, spend 20 minutes on quadriceps, 20 minutes on hamstrings and calves, and 20 minutes of speed walking. (On this "leg day," you may want to walk first since you may find it too difficult to walk after working legs.) On Day 2, spend 20 minutes on shoulders, 20 minutes on chest, and 20 minutes speed walking. On Day 3, work lats for 20 minutes then work lower back and abdominals for 20 minutes and then aerobics for 20. On Day 4, work biceps for 20, triceps for 20 and cardiovascular for 20. Day 5 you start all over again.

This is basically the routine I follow year-round. Remember that it is the intensity of your workout that counts, not the amount of time you spend in the gym. I utilize a lot of supersets and giant sets. For instance, when I work my quads, I do a set of front squats, back squats, leg presses and thigh extensions all in a row with no rest in between and going nearly to failure at each set. This is exhausting but extremely effective. Doing four sets of these in 20 minutes is a very good way to develop your legs.

Four-Day Per Week Workout

MONDAY AND THURSDAYS:

4   x 10 Squat
3   x 10 Stiff-legged dead lift (feet on box so that the bar touches the top of your feet)
3   x 10 Seated calf raises
3   x 20 Standing calf raises
4   x 10 Lat pulls
4   x 10 Lat rows
3   x 10 Standing curls
3   x 10 Seated curls

TUESDAYS AND FRIDAYS:

4   x 10 Bench presses
4   x 10 Incline bench presses
4   x 10 Seated behind the neck military presses
3   x 10 Standing upright rows
4   x 10 Pushdown triceps presses
3   Sets leg lifts
3   Sets crunches for abdominals (to failure)

On Wednesdays and Saturdays do aerobic exercises. Rest on Sundays.

There are several variations of advanced workouts that I will discuss. These include the Three-on and One-off, where you work legs on day one; chest/shoulders/triceps on day two; back/lats/biceps/abs on day three; rest on day four. Then start the cycle over again.

An example of Four-on and One-off would be Quadriceps/Calves on day one; Chest/Shoulders on day two; Hamstrings (stiff legged dead lifts and leg curls)/Lats on day three; day four would be Biceps/Triceps/Calves; take day five off; then start over again.

These latter two workouts would be for advanced lifters seeking to train each muscle group with great intensity for a period of about 20 minutes per muscle, utilizing from 9 to 16 sets per body part, and also doing supersets where you do, for instance, standing curls and then seated curls without any rest in between sets. Or do giant sets, which are what I use for maximum leg development, where you might do a set of 12 squats and then immediately do 10 or 12 hack squats, then 10 or 12 leg presses, then 10 or 12 thigh extensions. Four of these giant sets are a great leg workout, or for any body part for that matter. Each time I do this, I work out with such intensity that I go right to the point of nearly losing my breakfast! These workouts develop good size, definition, and moderate strength. On the other hand, to develop greater strength you would do pyramid sets, starting off with a set of 12 reps for warm-up, then going to a set of 10, set of 8, set of 6, set of 4, using a heavier and heavier weight, and resting anywhere from two to five minutes between sets. This particular workout would be used primarily to develop strength. It is a good idea when doing these advanced routines to change your routine every two or three months. It is OK to use different exercises for each workout to keep your body from becoming accustomed, which oftentimes keeps your body from making progress. Remember especially in the advanced workouts, it is not how much time you put in a gym that counts, it is what you do while you are there.

If you work with great intensity, 20 minutes is enough for any body part. Only when you are trying to develop greater power and rest longer between sets while you are doing low repetitions would you need to work more than 20 minutes per body part. Therefore, you can count on a maximum lifting time of one hour each day and still make tremendous gains.

High School Athlete Lifting Routine

Monday: LEGS
Squats 4 x 10 Hack squat 4 x 10 Thigh curls 4 x 10
Standing calves 3 x 10 Seated calves 3 x 30

Tuesday: PUSH
Bench press 4 x 10 Incline bench press 4 x 10
Behind neck press 4 x 10 Upright rows 3 x 10
Close-grip bench 3 x 10 Push-downs 3 x 10

Wednesday: PULL
Lat pull-down 4 x 10 Lat rows 4 x 10 Standing curls 4 x 10 Dumbbell curls 4 x 10 Crunches for abdominals
Neck

Thursday: Front squat 4 x 10 Thigh extension 4 x 10 Calves 6 x 30
Stiff-legged dead lifts on box

Friday: SAME AS TUESDAY

Saturday: Power clean 4 x 10 Lat pulls 4 x 10 Standing curls 4 x 10 Seated curl 4 x 10 Crunch
Neck

Sunday: REST

Children and Weightlifting

As I travel around the country doing weightlifting exhibitions, one of the questions I am most frequently asked is, "At what age should my child begin lifting weights, and is it harmful?" There are many myths about weightlifting and children lifting weights. Most of them, erroneous as they may be, really cloud the issue. Weightlifting is merely a form of exercise that is specifically pointed towards taxing the skeletal muscle system.

Any pediatrician would say exercise is necessary for the child to be healthy. As far as what age to begin, it's not unusual to read about an infant learning how to swim before he can walk. I believe any child from the age of three and over, can benefit through a moderate weightlifting program. It helps build a young person's self-esteem as he/she learns to appreciate his/her body, and it also enhances his/her God-given abilities. It strengthens his/her ability to compete in sports and other activities with his/her peers and can have a very wholesome, beneficial effect. However, there are precautions that should be taken, as in any sport.

The main caution is to make sure that any time a child is doing either bench presses or squats, he has a spotter. This person should have enough strength to take the weight off the child and set it down safely, in case the child were to stumble, slip or perhaps not be able to complete the lift. When supervised, weight training is as safe as any other sport or activity that most healthy children participate in.

It is a difficult task to hold the interest level of a young person on any one thing for a long duration. I believe that a simple and less time-consuming routine will keep the child from "burning out" and help him stay on this program. I recommend four 30-minute sessions each week. These would consist of doing upper body exercises on Tuesdays and Fridays. This amount of time would be enough to achieve desired results and effects and to encourage the child by his own accomplishments to continue in his training. As far as how much weight the child should use, that can be easily determined by allowing the child, in each particular exercise (the bench press, for instance), to take a weight that he can lift 10 times comfortably. If the child is quite small, then you might want to start with as little as 10 or 15 lbs. and then graduate from there. One thing most kids concern themselves with is how much they can do in comparison with their friends. It is very important that the child realizes from the beginning that what is important is his own personal advancement in gaining strength and muscular weight and not the amount of weight for his size. However, as with any other sport, some kids have a little more natural ability than others do. In weightlifting this natural ability does not begin to emerge as drastically until adolescence. Regardless, the child should be encouraged to stick with the weight he can do comfortably and progress with it at his own speed.

Because of the lack of hormonal maturity, a child will not progress nearly as rapidly (even percentage wise) as his adult counterpart. Even though results will be obvious and well worth the time as a strong foundation is built, expectations of tremendous gains in strength might prove to be frustrating rather than an advantage. Also, until the age of 12 or 13, girls will be able to do exactly the same routine that boys are doing if they, for whatever the reason, desire to increase their strength. They should be able to progress as well as boys and, in some cases, may even be stronger as a result of their earlier physical maturity.

Chapter Six

SPECIAL PURPOSE DIETS

The Low Carbohydrate Lifetime Program

First, it must be acknowledged that if you are overweight, you are not greedy, not weak-willed, not lazy, not self indulgent, not awful, but in all probability, metabolically unfortunate. Being fat is not an accidental accumulation of extra ounces. It is a basic metabolic disorder related to ill health. Food compulsion is not a character disorder. It is a chemical disorder called hyperinsulinism. A person with hyperinsulinism is "carbohydrate sensitive," meaning they are truly addicted to carbohydrates (especially sugar).

This metabolic disorder called hyperinsulinism causes your body to produce radical amounts of insulin when you consume a diet high in sugar and refined carbohydrates. Insulin is the single most significant determinant of your weight. Insulin is the fat producing hormone. When a person with hyperinsulinism eats carbohydrates, the body dumps huge amounts of insulin in the blood stream, leaving a constant sensation of hunger that can only be satiated by constant overeating, creating a vicious cycle.

But take heart! There is hope! The bypassing of carbohydrates is our ultimate solution. Protein and fats produce almost no change in your insulin level. The metabolic defect of hyperinsulinism can be circumvented by restricting carbohydrates. The Low Carbohydrate Lifetime Program allows you to lose weight while actually eating a higher number of calories than you were before starting the program. And, if you choose to eat fewer calories, you'll lose weight very fast. This plan is so effective at dissolving fat that it can create fat loss greater than occurs in fasting.

Here are some more great attributes of this program:
- No limit is set on the amount of food you can eat.
- No willpower is needed because there is no hunger.
- It is safe, luxurious, and state-of-the-art.
- It restores your vigor and health.
- It includes very rich foods.
- It produces steady weight loss.

So how do you lose weight quickly, easily, and without much pain or bother? How do you lose pounds and inches and keep them off—all hunger free? First let's examine three types of people who need this diet. See which category you fit in:

1) This person doesn't overeat. In fact, he eats less than most of his friends. But he still cannot lose weight, and sometimes gains. He often says, "I'm really very disciplined—it must be my metabolism."

THIS PERSON TRULY DOES HAVE A METABOLIC PROBLEM.

2) This person is obsessed with food and binges often. Late night eating is a habit. He craves sweets, breads, or high carbohydrate foods. He will nibble all day if food is available. He eats compulsively. He is moody, depressed, irritable, and has bouts of fatigue. He always seems to be hungry. He may feel better briefly after eating a food he craves.

THIS PERSON HAS GLUCOSE INTOLERANCE.

3) Some people have a single food craving or food-group craving.

THESE PEOPLE HAVE A FOOD ADDICTION OR FOOD ALLERGY.

Here are some very important pre-diet steps: 1) Stop taking any unnecessary medications. 2) Get a medical checkup. 3) Get a blood test to determine your cholesterol, triglyceride, glucose, insulin, and uric acid.

There are FOUR stages of the LOW-CARBOHYDRATE PROGRAM:

1) THE CORRECTIVE DIET (14 Days)
2) THE CONTINUED WEIGHT LOSS DIET
3) THE PRE-MAINTENANCE DIET (Last 10 pounds)
4) THE LIFETIME MAINTENANCE PROGRAM

The CORRECTIVE DIET contains, for all practical purposes, zero carbohydrates. It forces your body into Ketosis/Lipolysis (Ketosis for short). Ketosis is explained shortly.

The CONTINUED WEIGHT LOSS DIET very gradually adds carbohydrates to your diet (for a maximum of 40 grams) but still keeps you in Ketosis.

The PRE-MAINTENANCE DIET is for losing your last 10 pounds and re-introduces you to more carbohydrates.

The LIFETIME MAINTENANCE PROGRAM lifetime plan.

What is Ketosis? It is the chemical proof that your body is consuming its own stored fat. In Ketosis you are in the fat-dissolving state, which is the most efficient path ever devised for getting you slim. The more ketones you release, the more fat you have dissolved. The burning of fat in the absence of dietary carbohydrates is a natural mechanism of our bodies— it's what sustains hibernating animals. Also, researchers note that brain tissue utilizes ketones more readily than glucose, making ketone bodies the "preferred fuel" for the brain.

Once you reach ketosis, losing weight becomes painless and hunger free. After the first 48 hours, ketosis suppresses hunger and lowers appetite. Ketosis is better than fasting; when you fast your body burns fat and muscle for energy. However, on a high protein ketogenic diet, virtually no muscle tissue is lost, only fatty tissue.

A word now about fat. The ease of getting into deep ketosis is based on the ratio of fat to carbohydrates. Studies show that by eating foods such as bacon, whipped heavy cream (with "Equal," no sugar added), cream cheese, mayonnaise, and other high fat, low carbohydrate foods, people were able to lose fat almost twice as fast as when they ate nothing at all! In the absence of carbohydrates, eating fat accelerates the burning of stored fat! Fat satiates the appetite and stops carbohydrate craving. It seems that fat has been getting a bad rap.

It must be noted that the biggest source of real health improvements gained from this diet comes from the excluding the typically huge consumption of junk carbohydrates, especially sugar and refined, highly processed foods.

Now let's get started!

THE CORRECTIVE DIET

This first stage contains basically zero carbohydrates and lasts only for two weeks. The only carbohydrates you eat are three loosely packed cups of salad per day (which can be divided to provide a small salad for lunch and one for dinner). This diet is purposely unbalanced in order to correct an unbalanced metabolism. It is not a lifetime regimen. What you will be doing is forcing your body into ketosis/lipolysis (meaning your body will be burning its own fat for fuel). If you are hungry, eat as much as you want, as long as it contains no carbohydrates.

For these first two weeks, you can lose anywhere from 8 to 15 pounds, but the average is somewhat less. If you are a rare person who does not lose on this diet, you must get more exercise and restrict the quantity of your daily food intake.

RULES OF CORRECTIVE DIET
- NO MORE THAN 20 GRAMS OF CARBOHYDRATES A DAY (allows for approximately 3 cups of salad vegetables, loosely packed)
- ADJUST FOOD QUANTITIES TO YOUR APPETITE
- ABSOLUTELY NO FORBIDDEN FOODS

What you may eat:
- ALL MEATS: BEEF, FISH, FOWL, PORK, LAMB, VEAL, VENISON, SHELLFISH, ETC.
- ALL EGGS
- VERY SMALL AMOUNTS OF CHEESES (NO DIET CHEESE, NO CHEESE SPREADS, NO WHEY CHEESES)
- SALAD VEGGIES INCLUDE LETTUCE, CUCUMBER, RADISHES, PEPPERS, CELERY, MUSHROOMS, OLIVES, BROCCOLI
- SALAD GARNISHES: BACON, SMALL AMOUNT OF GRATED CHEESE, EGG
- HIGH FAT SALAD DRESSINGS WITH NO SUGAR ADDED (SUCH AS BLUE CHEESE)

- SPICES: ALL, BUT NONE WITH SUGAR
- BEVERAGES: NOTHING WITH SUGAR, NOTHING WITH CALORIES, NOTHING WITH CARBOHYDRATES. ONLY ARTIFICIAL SWEETENERS (SWEET-N-LOW OR EQUAL)
- COFFEE CAN HAVE SMALL AMOUNT OF CREAM (HALF-AND-HALF)
- BUTTER (not margarine), VEGTABLE OILS, MAYONNAISE, THE FAT PART OF MEAT AND FOWL

What's not allowed:
- NO SORBITOL, MANNITOL, HEXITOL, OR ANY SWEET-ENER ENDING WITH THE LETTERS "-OSE," SUCH AS FRUCTOSE
- AVOID SUGARLESS GUM—IT HAS CARBOHYDRATES!
- AVOID COUGH SYRUPS AND COUGH DROPS FILLED WITH SUGARS
- AVOID SAUCES MADE WITH CARBS (SUCH AS SUGAR)
- AVOID BREADING ON YOUR MEAT
- AVOID FLOUR AS A THICKENER (USED IN MOST GRAVIES)
- AVOID HAMBURGERS WITH BREADING MIXED IN
- NO FRUITS, STARCHES, GRAINS, SUGAR, JUNK FOODS, REFINED CARBOHYDRATES (SUCH AS WHITE FLOUR), MILK, WHITE RICE, MARGARINE, HONEY, POTATO STARCH

TIP:

YUMMY DESSERT: Sugar free Jello with one tablespoon whipped heavy cream to which Equal has been added (No sugar).

TREAT: Coffee with equal, couple of tablespoons of half and half and whipped heavy cream.

SNACKS: 1 oz. Nuts (macadamia nuts are lowest in carbs), cheese, pickles, fried pork skins.

Some sample meals on the Corrective Diet include:

Cheese omelet, chicken salad with real mayonnaise, chopped sirloin, olives, deviled eggs (no sweet pickle relish), nuts, ham and eggs, tuna fish salad, pork chops, steak, lobster with pure butter (not margarine), pot roast. Sounds great, doesn't it?

You must take the following SUPPLEMENTS daily:

Very broad Multiple Vitamin

Vitamin C (2000 mg.)

Vitamin E (800 I.U.)

Beta Carotene (25,000 I.U.)

Chromium picolinate (400-600 mcg.)

To confirm you are in ketosis and that your fat is melting away, use the "Ketostix," which can be found in most larger drug stores and is usually by diabetic supplies. After two days on the Corrective Diet, check urine stream with "Ketostix" every two to three hours for a couple of days to find when you get your darkest purple reading. Then you need only check for ketosis at this critical time of day when you are on the Corrective Diet and the Continued Weight Loss Diet.

HAVE FAITH—in the absence of carbohydrates, the body has no choice but to burn its own fat. Remember, the ease of getting into deep ketosis is based on the ratio of fat to carbohydrates so strive for maximum amount of fat for the first two-week correction diet.

You'll still have an appetite, but the days of obsession are gone! The 14 day Corrective Diet does the following:

- Switches your body from carbo-burning to fat-burning
- Stabilizes your blood sugar
- Stops cravings through abstinence, not moderation
- Breaks addictive eating patterns

EXERCISE

Exercise aerobically 30 minutes at least 4 times a week. Walking is considered an aerobic exercise if you are walking fast enough so that you sweat.

Anaerobic exercise (weight lifting) builds muscle and makes it easier to maintain ideal weight. Keep in mind that your ideal weight may be somewhat higher with a muscular body, because muscle weighs more than fat. A good rule of thumb would be a total body workout three days a week for 30 minutes. For instance, lift weights on Monday, Wednesday, and Friday. Exercise aerobically on the other days.

THE CONTINUED WEIGHT LOSS DIET

After you have completed the first 14 days on the Corrective Diet, you should begin the Continued Weight Loss Diet. You should stay on this diet until you come within 10 pounds of your ideal weight. You will still need to remain in Ketosis during this stage as you gradually increase your carbohydrates by 5 grams every two weeks. The maximum grams of carbohydrates you should work up to is 40 grams. Keep checking your "Ketostix" once a day. Stay purple, or you will have to start all over again with the Corrective Diet.

On the Continued Weight Loss Diet, the only carbs you are allowed are moderate helpings of low-carbohydrate vegetables and salads. You will definitely need to use the carbohydrate gram counter in this book to determine which vegetables and salads have approximately 5 grams of carbohydrates.

Most people find that after a couple of weeks on this diet, urges to eat sweets and starches totally disappear! After a month on this diet, for most people, sweets and starchy foods no longer fill a spot in one's imagination.

Constipation may be a problem. You may use a gentle laxative occasionally. Also, remember to include high-fiber vegetables in your allotment of carbohydrates. Some examples of good fiber vegetable sources are broccoli and cabbage. Try to work up to 25 grams of fiber daily. Our fiber chart will be useful.

Remember, your weight loss is proportional to your exclusion of carbohydrates. As you go up the carbohydrate scale at the rate of five additional grams every two weeks, you will eventually reach a number where you stop losing weight. Back off to the preceding level of carbohydrates. This is your Critical Carbohydrate Level (CCL).

Everybody hits plateaus (periods where no weight comes off). The first few times you hit a plateau almost never represents your CCL. To identify your CCL, you must make sure you are losing neither pounds nor inches for several weeks. Often, when the scales show no weight loss, you are losing inches. Sometimes too much salt can make you hold water, which can deceive the scales as to your progress.

Your "Ketostix" still has to be purple during this Continued Weight Loss Diet, even if only slightly so. The purple reading, along with your continued weight loss indicates you are still in that wonderful "fat burning" state.

THE PRE-MAINTENANCE DIET

When you get to within the last 10 pounds of your ideal weight, you will begin the Pre-Maintenance Diet. Now is the time to take things a little bit slower. Plan on losing your last 10 pounds over 2 to 3 months. Ideally, you should increase carbohydrates until your are losing less than a pound a week.

On the Pre-Maintenance Diet, you'll learn what exceptions you can make while still losing weight slowly. Start with one deviation per week, such as one fruit or one baked potato. However, by the time you reach your goal weight, you might be enjoying three such deviations per week, as long as you are still losing and not gaining weight. (The "Ketostix" does not play a part at this stage of the program.)

WARNING: Without Ketosis, the wonderful advantage of appetite suppression goes away. If carbohydrate cravings return, you can cure them with several days of the Corrective Diet. Another warning: Many people get into trouble during this stage of the program because they don't recognize just how strict their diets must remain.

The Low Carbohydrate Lifetime Program actually involves using all four stages of the diet when appropriate.

THE LIFETIME MAINTENANCE PROGRAM

The Lifetime Maintenance Program begins when you reach your ideal weight. It must be stressed that the average person must stay between 40 to 60 grams of carbohydrates daily for the rest of his life if he is to remain healthy and trim. Cautiously reintroduce vegetables, as well as whole grains such as oats, barley, wild rice, and buckwheat. Even an occasional potato and fruit a day are permissible.

Basically, this lifetime program includes most vegetables, nuts, seeds, some grains and starches (to the extent that your metabolism allows so that no weight gain takes place), and occasional fruit. Also, some high-fat foods like butter and cream can be used. A good plan would include something like two potatoes weekly, with the only other carbohydrates being low-carbohydrate vegetables and salads (and plenty of them).

Most fruits are high in natural sugars and will always be somewhat risky for you to consume. Restrict your consumption of sweets made with real sugars to the very occasional slice of birthday or wedding cake, but BEWARE! Remember the awful state you were in before you began your road to health. You may arouse the sleeping demon if you go back to eating foods that you once craved.

Get on the scale daily. If you've gone five pounds or more over your ideal weight, you must start the Corrective Diet to lose all the weight you've regained before beginning the Lifetime Maintenance Program again. The Corrective Diet will jump-start your metabolism only until maximum Ketosis takes place, as evidenced by a full measure of appetite suppression.

If you binge, binge on protein/fat foods. Be endlessly wary of sugar, corn syrup, white flour, corn starch, and pre-packaged junk food. Use caffeine in moderation. Remember, addictions can only be managed through abstinence.

A final footnote is the importance of lots of pure, fresh water. For optimal health, drink eight 8-ounce glasses of water a day.

In summary, those people who are committed to following the low-carbohydrate program for a lifetime have little or no difficulty maintaining their ideal weight. Dieting success on a properly managed, low-carbohydrate diet is almost unavoidable. The best rule of thumb for the rest of your life is never to allow yourself to be more than five pounds above your ideal weight.

The Fruit, Fish and Fowl Diet

This is a very simple and healthy diet. There are no restrictions on the amount of food you can eat. However, what is always important to us is common sense. On this diet, you may eat all the non-fried fish, chicken, and turkey that you like, and also egg whites. Here is the sample menu:

Breakfast
5 or 6 scrambled egg whites or Egg-Beaters
1 slice non-buttered wheat toast
Grapefruit

Lunch
Broiled chicken (no buttery sauces)
Fruit (unlimited)

Supper
Roasted turkey
Fruit (unlimited)

Make sure that you eat some white meat or egg whites at each meal and one or two pieces of fruit also. Fruit as an in-between meal snack is good. You may substitute a vegetable for lunch or supper if there is no butter or oil of any kind used in its preparation.

In essence this diet gives you a variety of foods to eat, but keeps you under 15 grams of fat per day. It is very important that you drink lots of water

This simple and easy diet is very effective.

Modified Liquid Diet

Some people have a very difficult time cutting back portions and types of food. For these people, a liquid diet can be a practical tool in getting you where you want to be. However, it is only used for a short period of time because the problem with most people who lose a lot of weight on a liquid diet is that they generally gain the weight back. So what I propose is a modified liquid diet where you get your fats and proteins primarily through liquid. However, you get some fiber and carbohydrates through fruit and salad.

Rather than going on a starvation formula of under 600 calories a day, which some liquid diets do, my recommendation is that you multiply your desired weight by 10, giving you the number of calories that you can consume. Ten would be the maximum; five would be the minimum. For instance, if you would like to end up weighing 120 pounds, then you would want to consume approximately 1200 calories per day. The minimum practical amount that you would want to go to would be 7.5 times your desired weight. If your goal were 120 you would consume 900 calories per day. At 50% you would consume 600 calories per day. My suggestion would be to start off at the 10:1 ratio and as long as you are losing 2-3 pounds per week, stay there! If after two weeks you plateau, then decrease to 7.5:1. Remember to never go under the 5:1 ratio. For instance, if you are a very large person and your desired weight is 200 pounds, then the 10:1 ratio would be 2000 calories per day, the 7.5:1 ratio would be 1500 calories per day, and the 5:1 ratio would be 1000 calories per day. A reasonable goal for fat loss is 1% of your start weight per week.

Regardless of your size, I would stick with somewhere between 500 – 1500 calories per day. With the ratio of 50% high quality protein, 25-30% low glycemic carbohydrates, and 20-25% high quality fat that would come from either flaxseed oil or olive oil. The carbohydrates would come from fruit and salad with vinegar and oil dressing. You could substitute some of the protein for grilled chicken salad, which generally would have approximately 20 grams of protein. To figure the percentages, the number of grams of each macronutrient needed, remember that carbohydrates and proteins have four calories per gram, and fats have nine calories per gram. So if you started on 1000 calories per day, 500 calories would come from protein, which would give you 125 grams a day. twenty-two grams of fat, which is 200 calories then 300 calories would come from carbohydrates, which is 75 grams per day. Use the nutritional chart in this book to give you a close guideline of what you need. The following is a sample diet of a 1000 calorie modified liquid diet.

Breakfast would consist of a whey and soy protein shake with one scoop each, giving you approximately 35 grams of protein mixed in water with one teaspoon of sugar free chocolate flavor and one tablespoon flaxseed or olive oil. Also, you can eat two pieces of dry wheat toast and your vitamin and mineral supplements taken with the milkshake and food. Supplementation is very important in this diet. The wheat toast should be a forty-calorie per slice bread. This should be your morning meal. At 10:00 a.m. eat a banana. At lunch, eat a salad with grilled chicken. At 3:00 p.m. eat one apple. At dinner eat grilled chicken salad. The salad may have tomatoes, broccoli, peppers, onions, and oil and vinegar for dressing, with four ounces of grilled chicken mixed in.

It is very important on this diet that you drink plenty of liquid, specifically at least ½ gallon (preferably one gallon) of water every day. The last meal would be the protein shake with no oil. This will give you approximately 120-125 grams of protein per day, 75-80 grams of carbohydrates, and 20 grams of fat. This totals to approximately 1000 calories per day.

To review, you have two shakes, one first thing in the morning with 2 slices of 40 calorie toast (dry) and one as your evening snack, two pieces of fruit, two salads, and along with the vitamin supplementation, you really do have very adequate nutrition. This also includes approximately 25 grams of fiber.

In conclusion, stay on this diet as long as you are losing weight. This is a diet I would advise to do under the care of a physician. It should pull weight off of you rapidly, especially if you are exercising, and doing resistance and aerobic training, along with this nutrition program. As you reach your desired weight, slowly reintegrate other foods, gradually increasing your calories, but not to the point that you gain back the unwanted pounds. This should get you where you want to be as quickly as possible.

Diet for Gaining Weight

The need to gain weight is only a problem that a small percentage of the population has. However, it is a serious problem for someone who really wants to gain weight for athletic purposes. I recommend that an athlete follow these guidelines:

- Get a minimum of one gram of protein per pound of body weight. A 200 pound athlete should get at least 200 grams or more of protein, Get all the carbohydrates that you can eat, while continuing to keep your fats moderately low. A rule of thumb to follow is to get between 20 and 30 calories per pound of your ideal weight. (Someone wanting to weigh 200 pounds would get between 4000 and 6000 calories per day.) The more active you are, the more calories you need. Your carbohydrates should come from complex carbs as much as possible, like pasta and vegetables.
- Eat $1/2$ pound red meat daily until you get to your desired weight, then cut back.
- Eat every 2 or 3 hours while awake.
- Consider high-calorie foods such as peanut butter. Peanut butter, when consumed with milk, makes an excellent source of protein.

- Snack an hour before you go to bed. A good snack would be a milkshake, made with ice milk, egg, milk, flavoring, banana or other fruit if desired.
- Get plenty of sleep.

As you are gaining weight, give yourself the pinch test. Pinch the skin on your abdomen to make sure you can't pinch over an inch of fat. If you do, you will want to cut back on your calories, but keep the protein and carbs really high.

For difficult-to-gain individuals, I recommend just getting all the calories you can. You may have to resort to eating a lot of high-fat foods, such as ice cream, whole cheese, red meat, whole dairy products, high-sugar foods, desserts, etc. (It's a tough job but somebody's go to do it!). Seriously, there are some people, especially adolescents, who cannot gain weight any other way but by going on a very high-calorie diet.

Remember, you cannot stay on this high-fat diet forever. It is especially important that you get plenty of rigorous exercise to stimulate muscle growth, so that you put on the right kind of weight.

Tips And Secrets

Crash dieting works against weight loss by causing the metabolism to drop and by converting muscle protein to fuel. Since muscle tissue is the major factor in caloric expenditure, then the body requires fewer calories to sustain itself.

If you are overweight, it probably took years to get that way. Don't lose heart if it takes you more than a few months to lose your extra weight.

Every 10 pounds you gain may be associated with a 5 point rise in your cholesterol level.

Being even slightly overweight might make women far more vulnerable to heart disease. In an eight-year study of women, the leanest women suffered the fewest heart attacks. Mildly obese women suffered more heart disease.

Today's preparation determines tomorrow's achievement. To indulge is to bulge!

A little sugar and fat make you crave even more. Exercise prevents cravings from striking and can douse them once they spark!

Skipping meals to save calories may slow down your metabolic rate by 20 percent. Bypassing one meal may make you so hungry that you binge at the next.

Even some diet-friendly foods lose their low-cal status if you overindulge.

Eat small frequent meals. Eat breakfast like a king, lunch like a prince, and dinner like a pauper.

Reduce calories gradually in a cyclical fashion.

Weight train to increase metabolism and preserve lean body mass.

The longer you resist temptation, the stronger you become. You end up feeling better about yourself because the craving is no longer in control—you are!

On your weight-loss program:

    Set a specific goal.

    Set a time frame.

    Adopt a specific plan.

Don't try to change everything at once.

Plan for relaxation and rewards!

Do you ever get irritable when dieting? The Hunger Center in the brain secretes a hormone called glannin when you are hungry. This causes the irritablility. Eating six meals a day, spread out, and eating slowly will cure this.

SEVEN SECRETS OF SUCCESS

These principles are the secrets of success of the highly advertised weight-loss programs.

  1) High water

  2) High fiber

  3) Low fat and Low sugar

  4) Low to moderate calorie intake

  5) Daily exercise

6) Accountability

7) Encouragement

This book offers all of these, except the personal, weekly accountability and encouragement that a private trainer or counselor offers.

I can't help but be amused by advertisements that run a special by saying, "Sign up and lose your first 15 pounds for only $50." You really don't have to pay anybody. You are the one who changes your eating habits and does the exercise.

This book gives you all the information you need to get and stay fit. However, as a therapist, I realize the importance of regular accountability and encouragement. If you feel the need for this, try the "Buddy" system. It ultimately depends on you, but having one or more friends that you meet with on a regular basis can help. Encourage each other, weigh each other, and hold each other to the fire in a kind manner. Don't accept excuses, and offer enthusiastic praise for each small success.

By the way, the important thing is to succeed. If you can't do it on your own, it is certainly OK to use a personal trainer or nutritional counselor. A good health club should have a program that can help, too.

Chapter Seven

SUPPLEMENTATION

Always take Vitamins and Minerals with a Meal

Vitamin and Mineral Supplementation

As in other fields of nutrition, there is much controversy regarding the need for vitamin and mineral supplementation. Some recommend megadoses of vitamins and minerals daily. Others disagree wholeheartedly with this. Some claim high doses of vitamin C keep you free of disease, and the anti-oxidants (C, E, and A) retard the aging process. This is fairly new research, but with some convincing evidence. There are those in the medical profession who are great proponents of vitamin supplementation for both mental and physical reasons.

I believe it is healthy and reasonable to take vitamins. Do you realize how many oranges, tomatoes, or strawberries you would have to eat to get 20 grams of vitamin C? (Suffice it to say you would have to start fairly early and binge the rest of the day to obtain that much.) Don't go overboard, and what your body does not use will be excreted.

I recommend that the average person take a large multi-vitamin-mineral tablet (morning); 1000 mg vitamin C (morning and evening); 10,000 units beta-carotene (morning only); and 200 to 400 units of vitamin E (morning and evening). Also, too much vitamin C can cause diarrhea.

You and your physician and nutritionist should be the judge of any radical supplementation program in which you wish to engage. If you would like a more aggressive supplement list, there is one following entitled Supplementation for Health Repartitioning (exchanging fat for muscle) and Youthful Longevity.

Vitamins and Minerals

Here is a listing of vitamins, the recommended daily allowance, and the foods where they are found.

VITAMIN A: Keeps the skin healthy. Helps in the functioning and maintenance of healthy eyes, skin, gums, hair, teeth, mucous membranes, and digestive tract. Also aids in the promotion of growth. **RDA:** 5,000 I.U. **WHAT FOODS SUPPLY IT?** Liver, dark green and deep yellow vegetables (broccoli, collards, carrots, pumpkin, sweet potatoes, winter squash, tomatoes, apricots, cantaloupe, strawberries, watermelon, butter, fortified margarine.

VITAMIN D: Necessary for the promotion of necessary growth in bone and teeth. Helps form bony tissue and cartilage. RDA: 400 I.U. WHAT FOODS SUPPLY IT? Butter, egg yolk, liver, fatty fish, fortified margarine, and milk. Vitamin D is also produced in the skin with stimulus of sunlight.

VITAMIN E: Protects the red blood cells from oxidation. Facilitates the effectiveness of Vitamin B-12. RDA: 30 I.U. WHAT FOODS SUPPLY IT? Meats and green vegetables contain small amounts. Whole-grain cereals and peanuts. Fortified and polyunsaturated oils of vegetable products, safflower oil.

VITAMIN C: (Absorbic Acid) Essential role in tooth and bone formation. Aids in wound healing. Helps in use and absorption of iron. RDA: 60 mg. WHAT FOODS SUPPLY IT? Broccoli, cabbage, tomatoes, green leafy vegetables, cantaloupe, grapefruit, oranges, strawberries.

VITAMIN (B1): Necessary for the normal functioning and growth of nerve tissue. Promotes good digestion and appetite. Assists body cells obtain energy by promoting adequate metabolism of sugar. RDA: 1.5 mg. WHAT FOODS SUPPLY IT? Whole-grain and enriched breads, cereals, potatoes, organ meats, pork, poultry, fish, other meats, milk, green vegetables, dried peas, and beans.

VITAMIN (B2): Aids in keeping the eyes healthy. Also helps keep skin around the nose and mouth healthy. Functions in the body's use of carbohydrates, fats, and proteins, specifically to release energy to cells. RDA: 1.7mg. WHAT FOODS SUPPLY IT? Milk, liver, lean meat, kidney, heart, egg enriched and whole-grain enriched breads and cereals.

NIACIN (B3): Plays role in normal respiration. Promotes maintenance of healthy skin. Aids in the release of energy to cells. RDA: 20 mg. WHAT FOODS SUPPLY IT? Fish, poultry, lean meat, peanut butter, peanuts, fish, peas, and whole-grain and enriched breads and cereals.

VITAMIN (BI2): Essential for the normal growth of red blood cells. Promotes normal functioning of all body cells. RDA: 6 mg. WHAT FOODS SUPPLY IT? Fish, meat, liver and other organ meats, eggs, shellfish, milk, cottage cheese, and other milk products, with the exception of butter

IRON: An essential ingredient of hemoglobin, the substance that enables red blood cells to carry oxygen throughout the body. RDA: 18 mg. WHAT FOODS SUPPLY IT? Kidney, heart, liver, oysters, lean meat, egg yolks, dried beans, dried peas, dark leafy green vegetables, dried fruit, breads.

CALCIUM: Enables blood to clot. Helps teeth and bones. Also required for activity of nerve and muscle cells. RDA: 1,000 mg. WHAT FOODS SUPPLY IT? Milk: fortified skim, low-fat, whole, buttermilk, cheeses made from skim or partially skim milk, (mozzarella), whole milk cheese (Cheddar), yogurt; leafy vegetables such as collards, dandelion kale, mustard, and turnip greens.

POTASSIUM: A component of lean body tissue. Helps to facilitate the growth and muscle strength. Helps to regulate acid-base and body water balance. Assists in maintaining neuro-muscular function. RDA: None. WHAT FOODS SUPPLY IT? Meats, milk, fruits, potatoes, and dark leafy green vegetables

MAGNESIUM: Activator of various enzymes. Aids in energy production and utilization, contraction of muscles and nerves, and building of tissue. RDA: 400 mg. WHAT FOODS SUPPLY IT? Bananas, dried beans, milk, most dark green leafy vegetables, whole-grain cereals, meats, nuts, peanuts and peanut butter.

ZINC: Activates various enzymes. A constituent of the hormone insulin. Facilitates healing of wounds and prevention of anemia, taste acuity. <u>RDA:</u> 15 mg. <u>WHAT FOODS SUPPLY IT?</u> Whole grains, dried beans and peas, shellfish (particularly oysters), cheese, meat and cocoa, nuts.

SODIUM: This is a key element in the regulation of acid base balance and water in the body. <u>RDA:</u> 150 mg. <u>WHAT FOODS SUPPLY IT?</u> Broth, gelatin dessert, table salt, baking soda, and most processed foods, some present in all natural foods.

SUPPLEMENTATION FOR HEALTH AND REPARTITION-ING AND YOUTHFUL LONGEVITY
Antioxidant and Anticarcinogenic

(FL = Fat Loss Specific)
(MG = Muscle Gain Specific)

Take with Meals:
Broad Multi-Vitamin and Mineral Tablet
Vitamin C: 2-6 grams ($^1/_2$ A.M.; $^1/_2$ P.M.)
Vitamin E: 800-1000 IU's (A.M.)
Beta-Carotene: 25,000 – 50,000 IU's (A.M.)
Acetyl L Carnitine: 500 mg A.M.
Aspirin: (A.M.)
Phyto Chem A.M.
Q10: 100 mg/day A.M.
DHEA (males: 50-100mg; Females 25-50 mg) (A.M.) FL;MG
Melatonin: 1-9 mg at bedtime
Chromium: 1000 mcg ($^1/_2$ A.M.; $^1/_2$ P.M.) FL
Garlic Odorless Capsules at Bedtime

Specific to Repartitioning:
C.L.A. (Conjugated Linoleic Acid) 6 – 750mg capsules
(two with each meal) FL; MG

Specific to Muscle Gain:
Vanadyl Sulfate: 50 mgs ($^1/_2$ A.M.; $^1/_2$ P.M.) FL; MG

Creatine Monohydrate immediately after workout: 20mgs for 5 days then 10 mgs daily mixed with Carb and Protein drink immediately after workout. MG

My only hesitation in adding in this section is my fear that many people will use it as the sole aspect of their program. It is the easiest of all to do, requiring only enough effort to purchase and then take some pills or powder. Please remember that, although you can attain results utilizing only any one section of this book, they alone can only take you so far.

(Note: We talked earlier about the importance of water in this program. Please keep that in mind [I almost added that portion of the text in this section; it is that important] that without water, your body can only function sub-optimally, particularly when taking supplements.)

Chromium picolinate

This micronutrient has often been touted as a miracle fat loss supplement. In fact, it functions to help maintain proper insulin levels in the body, and some anecdotal evidence indicates that it may help to lower cholesterol. A med-line review of studies done on chromium indicates that "chromium picolinate was ineffective in enhancing body fat reduction" in the experimental group. [J Sports Med Phys Fitness 1995 Dec;35(4):273-80]. Another study suggested that "routine chromium supplementation has no beneficial effects on body-composition change or strength gain in men." [Am J Clin Nutr 1996 Jun;63(6):954-65] If, however, you decide to give chromium a try, start with 400 mcg. per day. If you want to raise the dose, after a week take 400 mcg twice a day. Do NOT exceed 1000 mcg a day. This is a micro nutrient, and it is not supposed to be found in high doses in your body.

Citrimax

Also known as Hydroxy Citric Acid (HCA) and Garcinia Cambogia, Citrimax is espoused by some to inhibit the conversion of sugars and proteins into fat. There are also people who say that this herb acts as a natural hunger suppressant. At this time, no studies could be found to support these claims. However, if you wish to give it a try, the recommended dose is 250 mg of HCA taken three times a day half an hour before ameals.

Pyruvate

A naturally occurring intermediary product of the body's storage of sugars, pyruvate has been shown in a recent study to aid in fat loss in calorie (carbohydrate) deprived women. Past studies using very high doses of pyruvate (30 grams per day, which would make using pyruvate very expensive) showed a significant effect on aiding in fat loss and slowing down fat storage. A recent study showed that as little as six grams per day over a six week time period with 30 minutes of exercise done five days per week effected a significant result in fat loss. With no change in absolute body weight, the pyruvate group lost almost 5 lbs. of fat, added about 3.5 lbs. of muscle, and had a 12% decrease in percent body fat [Colker C, Stark R, Kaiman D, et al. The effects of a pyruvate based dietary supplement on weight loss, body composition, and perceived vigor and fatigue levels in mildly overfat individuals. Am J Clin Nutr 1997 (in press)]. The recommended dose is 2 grams taken three times a day with meals, or 3 grams taken twice with meals.

Thermogenic Formulas

This includes supplements that contain a combination of MaHuang or Ephedra (a plant that contains the chemical ephedrine HCL) and Guarana, Kola Nut, or Bissey Nut (plants that contain caffeine). The effectiveness of these products has recently been scientifically scrutinized in many studies. The result of these studies suggests that they are very effective in temporarily raising the metabolic rate of an individual. In other words, they effect a thermogenic response (raising the body's core temperature). The body uses fat to fuel this increase in body temperature, and therefore, thermogenics have been shown to be effective fat burners. Short-term use does have potential side effects, including shakiness, nervousness, headaches, insomnia, increased heart rate, etc. Studies suggest that these side effects will probably diminish over time. In general, you should consult a physician before initiating use of any supplement. Specifically, if you have high blood pressure, mitral valve prolapse, are pregnant, or taking MAO inhibitors, you should definitely consult your physician before taking these products. The recommended dose is 200 mg of caffeine with 20 mg of ephedrine, or 334 mg of MaHuang Extract with 910 mg of Guarana extract. You may decide to take this dose up to three times a day, spaced three to four hours apart. Common side effects are a burst of energy, shakiness, and trouble sleeping. Don't take this supplement after 4 p.m., or you might not be able to fall asleep!

L-Carnitine

Carnitine is used to break down the long chained triglycerides (fatty acids) so your body can more easily use them for energy. The average recommended dose is 500 mg three times a day on an empty stomach, and the preferred (and most expensive) source is acetyl-l-carnitine. There is, however, no scientific evidence that taking oral L-carnitine can aid weight loss. "Although there are some theoretical points favouring potential ergogenic effects of carnitine supplementation, there is currently no scientific basis for healthy individuals or athletes to use carnitine supplementation to improve exercise performance." [Sports Med 1996 Aug;22(2):109-32]

Other Aids

AMINO ACIDS

Amino acids in powder or tablet form referred to as "free

form acids" are simply that. They are a correct combination of amino acids usable for human consumption in building tissue. They are pure protein. Amino acids are not necessary if you have adequate protein in your diet. However, some body builders take three grams of amino acids with each meal to ensure they are getting usable complete protein. As I mentioned in the chapter on nutrition, the human body needs complete protein. If you are getting your protein from vegetable sources, and it's not complete, amino acids would be helpful in making the protein into a more usable form. Also, if you are not getting enough protein in your diet, amino acids are very helpful. But if you are, they are not necessary.

PROTEIN POWDER

Again, if you are getting enough protein in your diet, additional protein powder is not necessary. However, if you are on a restricted diet and you are not getting enough protein, then protein powder can help. Normally it comes with no fat and very little carbohydrates and can be an excellent source of protein for those on low calorie diets. It is important to understand that your body can use only so much protein. Normally you cannot use over 40 grams per sitting. Any more protein than your body uses is a waste of money and will not help you gain muscular weight. Protein in the body is needed to keep a positive nitrogen balance somewhere between 1/3 gram and 3/4 gram per pound of body weight depending on your muscle-to-fat ratio. The more muscular and the less fat percentage you have would dictate a need for a somewhat greater amount of protein. But any more than 1/2 gram per pound of body weight would probably not be used unless you are a hard-training strength athlete. Even then, one gram per pound of body weight would be adequate. This could probably be obtained through a regular diet. If you feel you are deficient, there are a number of good protein powders on the market in health food stores. Make sure you read the label to get the composition, and make sure it is complete with all the essential amino acids.

EVEN THOUGH THERE ARE AIDS THAT CAN BE HELPFUL IN REACHING YOUR DESIRED PHYSIQUE, NOTHING TAKES THE PLACE OF GOOD NUTRITION AND HARD WORKOUTS—NOTHING! GOOD NUTRITION AND HARD WORKOUTS, BY THEMSELVES ALONE, WILL BRING THE DESIRED RESULTS.

CAFFEINE

Caffeine is considered a drug that occurs naturally in more than 60 plants. It's found most prominently in coffee, tea, soft drinks, chocolate, analgesics containing aspirin as well as many over-the-counter diet aid products. Caffeine works as a stimulant to the central nervous system and helps mobilize various hormones that are involved in the metabolic process. It enhances muscle contraction and improves mobilization and utilization rate of fats and carbohydrates for energy. Too much caffeine, however, can be detrimental. Arnold Schwarzenneger, the world-famous body builder, for years has advocated drinking two cups of coffee before a workout. However, too much can cause you to be nervous and jittery. I also want to point out that I do this and recommend that others drink coffee before a workout, but let that be the only caffeine consumed for the day. Even though I enjoy soft drinks, there are a number on the market that have no caffeine, as well as decaffeinated coffees, etc. I also want to point out that scientific studies have shown that too much caffeine can lower testosterone levels, which will cause you to lose strength. So remember that even though I advocate small amounts of caffeine before workouts, that's the only time it should be used. Otherwise, it could contribute to hypertension, hyperactivity, nervousness, irritability, and other maladies. The best dose of caffeine is about 3 milligrams of caffeine per kilogram of body weight. Below that, little performance is noted, and any more than that can cause detriment to performance. Administering caffeine before athletic activity is most useful to those who don't consume caffeine at any other time. Improved uptake of fatty acids by the muscle cells and enhanced use of muscle triglycerides are responsible for the enhanced performance in endurance sports. The stimulation of the central nervous system causes you to be more alert and enhances the psyching up process for lifting or explosive power. Fat loss with exercise is increased with small amounts of caffeine taken one half hour before exercise. The half-life of caffeine, or the length of effectiveness lasts for two-three hours. If you have been advised against the use of caffeine by your physician, follow that advice. People with ulcers are cautioned against using caffeine because it causes hyperacidity levels, an increase up to 400% of acid level in the intestines.

INOSINE

Inosine is also a product that has come from Russian research. Russian weight lifters use this during intense workouts. This is available in most health food stores and 1/2 to 1 gram should be taken 30 minutes before a workout. Japanese researchers have classified inosine as a metabolic activator. Inosine belongs to the purine nucleoside group and can easily penetrate cell walls where it promoted ATP (adenosine triphosphate) production. ATP supplies energy to generate muscular contractions, to ignite nerve tissue, to maintain and repair body tissues, and to fuel energy transformations involved in reproduction and growth. It's an energy-rich compound that is stored in the cells of the body. Inosine stimulates the replacement of ATP, which is used during strenuous exercise. Inosine also takes a direct part in metabolizing sugar, and enhances the synthesis of protein as well.

GROWTH HORMONE RELEASERS

The use of amino acids arginine and ornithine promotes fat loss. They also serve in building muscle tissue through the use of stimulating growth hormone (GH). This must be used on an empty stomach 3-4 hours following the last meal, preferably right before bedtime and/or before peak-output strenuous exercise. These are the times your body naturally releases growth hormones. Growth hormone decreases naturally as you pass the age of 25. However, using these growth hormone stimulants or releasers that work by stimulating the pituitary gland to produce higher natural levels of growth hormone can cause re-enactment of growth hormone levels of people in their late teens. Diabetics should not use this because it tends to block correct insulin use. Normally one should take twice as much arginine as ornithine. Before going to bed you should take perhaps eight grams of arginine, four grams of ornithine.

A solid, deep sleep is very important for the release process of growth hormone. The effects of growth hormone are decreasing fat percentage and increasing muscle mass. We are what we are because of body chemicals. Women are women because of estrogen and men are men because of testosterone. However, the growth hormone has an equally stimulating effect on women as well as men. You would want to cut this dose in half before exercise. By the way, the stuff tastes horrible. If you take it in tablet form, which is easier on your stomach, you should take it 11/2 hours before exercise because the tablets take longer to dissolve. If you use the powder form, stir it up in water and drink it. The presence of B5, B6 and Vitamin C are important in the use of growth hormone releasers. Also, it is important to take multivitamin and mineral tablets perhaps four times the RDA to ensure the antitoxic effects of anti-aging effects that free radicals produce. Antitoxins are vitamin C and E. These are very important. Vitamin B6 especially augments exercise-induced GH release. Niacin, a form of B3, is a good GH releaser and helps to control blood sugar levels. A low glycemic index diet is also helpful. We are not prescribing that you do this; however, this is something some athletes are doing to increase their muscular mass as well as decrease body fat percentages. This is not a steroid you hear about in the news media. This is stimulating or manipulating your own body chemistry to develop enhanced amounts of growth hormone.

INOSITOL CHOLINE

Inositol has long been recognized for the role it plays in fat mobilization. It also can be converted to glucose by the human body. It can assist in maintaining blood glucose levels during dieting. Inositol is also known to reduce the ketosis that happens during severe dieting or prolonged intense exercise.

Choline plays important roles as well in metabolizing fat. The amount required above the amount synthesized by the body is in the unproven category even though much research is being done on this. Realizing that triglycerides are mobilized from fat cells, one possible way of decreasing body fat is by increasing its use as a fuel. In order to do this, other nutritional factors must be involved. Two of these necessary nutrients are inositol and choline. Having interviewed a number of top physique competitors, I found many of them take inositol and choline supplements to help decrease their fat percentage and give them what they call "a thinner skin" to increase the muscular definition.

GINSENG

Herbal remedies, such as ginseng, have long been touted in Far Eastern countries for their curative powers. The Soviets used Ginseng for its medical properties and claimed that daily doses used for 15-45 days increased physical endurance and mental work capacity Other researchers feel that ginseng works by increasing the efficiency of the adrenal and pituitary glands. However, overuse of ginseng can cause ginseng abuse syndrome, which can cause insomnia, nervousness, irritability, diarrhea, and rashes, or contribute to high blood pressure. Also, women are cautioned that estrogen-like compounds found in some ginseng can cause some breast tenderness, vaginal bleeding, and menstrual irregularities. But, when taken in moderation in the form of capsules and mild teas, ginseng appears to be safe and a mild stimulant.

There are two species of Ginseng-Korean (Panex ginseng or Panex schinseng) and Siberian (Elutherococcus senticoccus). The latter seems to be the most productive. A number of studies have shown ginseng to be effective as a training aid for raising the subject's mood as well as his endurance.

Injuries: How to Speed Healing

This chapter is not designed to replace your physician, who should be consulted whenever you have a questionable injury, ache or pain. However, there are standard treatments that certified trainers, chiropractors, and physicians use that do aid in the healing process.

The acronym R.I.C.E. is a standard term used by trainers to describe the way you initially handle an injury, which has an impact on the rate of healing. "R" stands for REST, which damaged tissues must have in order to heal. "I" stands for ICE. It is important to ice down an injury as quickly as possible, and then to use ice for the next 48 hours. "C" stands for COMPRESSION. Wrap the injury with an Ace bandage. However, if there is a possibility of a broken bone or if a muscle has completely torn loose, rush the injured person to a medical facility. "E" stands for ELEVATION. Elevate the injured limb above heart level.

ICE MASSAGE

This is a very effective means of decreasing pain in small areas where trauma may have occurred. Take an 8-oz. Styrofoam cup, and fill it ³/₄ with water. Freeze it. Peel the bottom off about 1 inch, exposing the ice. Massage the injured area for 3-5 minutes. The massage can be repeated once the temperature of the area returns to normal.

HEAT

Heat should be avoided in areas where inflammation is present, as it will increase local blood flow and could promote greater edema (swelling). However, when cold cannot be tolerated, using heat to decrease muscle guarding by decreasing pain my be appropriate. In this case, use heat for 3-5 minutes to decrease pain. Repeat several times per hour as needed.

HYDROTHERAPY WHIRLPOOL

Whirlpool, where the water temperature is approximately 104 degrees, may be helpful in decreasing pain and muscle guarding. Keep the treatment time to no more than 5 minutes.

ULTRASOUND

This deep heat modality (using sound waves to vibrate water molecules) is used clinically to decrease pain and guarding.

TENDINITIS

This is simply inflammation of a tendon. Over the counter anti-inflammatories such as aspirin and ketoprofen can be helpful in decreasing the amount of inflammation. Ice massage can also be helpful in decreasing pain and inflammation. Sometimes, in severe cases, medical attention may be necessary. Common treatments involve corticosteroids in the form of injections or pills.

MUSCLE STRAIN OR SPRAIN

This is when tearing of the tissue occurs, commonly from a traumatic injury. Most serious lifters experience this from time to time. Both of my pectoralis major (chest) muscles have been torn at least twice, causing the whole side of my chest to turn black and blue for up to two weeks. Ice massage and ultrasound helped my body heal quickly.

LOW BACK PAIN

This common ailment ranges in intensity from slight to severe. In cases with leg involvement (i.e. numbness, tingling or weakness), seek medical attention immediately. In less severe cases, over the counter anti-inflammatories, rest, modalities (such as ice or heat), and muscular re-education (see a qualified personal trainer) can be helpful in the recovery process.

MUSCLE SORENESS

Thought to be the product of micro-tears in the connective tissue of muscles, low intensity (light weight, higher repetition) exercise in a pain free range of motion can help tissues heal, and can increase circulation to those areas to flush out metabolic waste. Over the counter anti-inflammatories, brief icing/heating, and rest may speed up the recovery process.

SHIN SPLINTS

This is pain on the front of your lower leg (below the knee) usually caused by jarring while running on a hard surface. The treatments recommended above may help to speed healing. When you initiate the activity again, make sure you have the proper footwear, and are performing on an appropriate surface (i.e. a track).

In summary, the old concept of "No pain, no gain" is false. Pain is not a warning signal. Pain indicates the presence of trauma, and that trauma must be addressed appropriately. If the pain doesn't dissipate, or if it gets worse, stop your activity and seek medical attention. Getting in shape is a lot like getting a tan; start a little at a time and gradually build up. Remember, an ounce of prevention is worth a pound of cure!

Chapter Eight

FIT AFTER 40

The good news is: It is never too late to start a fitness program. People in nursing homes who have begun exercise programs have made miraculous gains in both bone and muscle density. As a matter of fact, research studies show that exercise is equally as important as—if not more important than—calcium in reducing the weakening affect of osteoporosis. Let me say that if you have been sedentary and relatively inactive, it is very important that you begin your exercise program slowly. Get a physical examination, including a complete blood profile, and discuss your fitness ambitions with your physician.

Again, start slowly. I would suggest a walking program on a daily basis, gradually building up 3 miles in 45 minutes. You'll be surprised at how quickly you will be able to reach this goal—normally within a month's time. Set yourself achievable goals, such as walking between 500 and 1000 miles per year—1000 miles would be approximately 3 miles per day, and 500 miles is approximately 1½ miles per day. Chart your progress.

Often I am asked what the best exercise is to get rid of the extra fat around the waist. People expect me to show them some type of sit-up or twist. However, the best exercise to trim the middle is brisk walking 2 to 3 miles every day. This burns fat tissue very effectively.

After you have built up your cardiovascular routine by walking 2 or 3 miles a day, I would then suggest that you spend 30 minutes 3 or 4 times per week doing exercises that stimulate the muscles in your entire body. Joining a health club would be practical. Get on a program where you work each muscle group twice a week. Example: Day 1, work legs (thigh, hamstrings, calves). Day 2, work chest, shoulders, triceps. Day 3 work lats, biceps, abdomen. Day 4, rest. Day 5, start all over again.

The ideal routine should take 30-60 minutes. You will be amazed at how much better you feel after you work your skeletal muscle system through weight training, and your lungs and heart through walking.

When you exercise, your body releases endorphins, causing joint pain to lessen and giving you an exhilarating attitude. It also provides you with a healthier outlook on life and much better health in general. Another advantage to weight training is that your body will take on a new shape, different proportions, you will stand more erect, and you will trade fat for muscle mass which will help burn more calories. You will end up with a much more pleasing shape an athletic, trim, firm body.

Remember, when beginning a weight training program, start slowly, doing just one set of each exercise the first workout. The next time, do two sets and gradually work up to three or four sets. This will help prevent some soreness.

The main thing to realize is that you can get into great shape after 40 years of age. Chris Dickerson never lifted weights in his life until he was 39-years-old. He went on to win the title of Mr. America after only three years of serious training. In my bodybuilding competition, I see men who are in their 50s and early 60s who have bodies of 25-year-olds. Many of them did not start until they were 40. So don't feel defeated before you start. There is a lot of potential in that body.

Most people don't want to become Mr. America, but just want to get in better shape. My neighbor is a nurse and a grandmother. She had high blood pressure and elevated cholesterol levels and was overweight. Within a year's time of walking briskly 45 minutes every evening, her blood pressure came down to low-normal, her pulse rate came down, and her cholesterol level dropped. After she began a low-fat diet (not counting calories but counting fat grams), her weight began to drop at a more rapid pace. Today she is much trimmer, feels great, and has a wonderful attitude. She is not the same person she was a year ago.

One of the keys to her success is her friend, Becky, and

Becky's husband. The three of them get out and have the best time briskly walking, enjoying a portion of every evening together. The companionship they share helps them to stay consistent, which in turn pays off in a healthier body. It will for you, too!

Chapter Nine

FITNESS AFTER RETIREMENT

Fitness After Retirement

Being involved in fitness for the last 25 years has given me the pleasure of seeing lots of friends grow old quite gracefully. These people who exercised in their 40s, and 50s, and 60s now have trim, fit, athletic-looking bodies while in their 70s.

There is nothing unusual about their success. I know some extremely strong men in their late 60s and early 70s who still compete in power lifting. And I know some bodybuilders who still compete on a national level in their 60s, who have always exercised and will never give it up because it is such a wonderful life-style.

But how about those who are in their retirement years and have never been on an exercise program. Some might say, "Well, I never have done it and it is too late to start now!" That couldn't be further from the truth. Exercising at any age will bring quick results. Don't be fooled by "Grandfather Time." As long as you can move, you can derive tremendous results from an exercise program.

As I mentioned before, studies done in nursing homes have shown that people derive great benefits from exercise at any age. In the retirement years, when schedules are more open, a regular weight lifting program is a great hobby! Also, weight lifting with light weights is a great way to rehabilitate muscles.

The guidelines I would suggest are: Consult a physician to get his approval. Start in moderation. Do something that you can enjoy and stick with, but make it a part of your everyday life. If you commit to 30 minutes or an hour a day, you will surely not only add years to your life, but also add a great deal of life to those years.

So don't wait any longer. Get started today on a program. Get out there and enjoy yourself!

Chapter Ten

SUMMARY

Finale-My 10 Tips

1. Drink a minimum of ¹/₂ gallon water daily.

2. Eat a minimum of 25 grams of fiber daily. If you are not currently doing this, gradually increase the fiber in your diet.

3. Walk or do some form of mild to rigorous exercise 30 minutes per day, every day.

4. Keep the amount of fats in your diet to below 25% (or under 25 grams) per day for consistent weight loss.

5. Don't use tobacco in any form.

6. Limit your intake of alcoholic beverages.

7. Limit your sugar intake.

8. Don't salt your food.

9. Keep your calorie intake to 10 times desired weight until you reach your goal.

10. After you have reached your goal, stick to a low-fat, low-sugar life-style and anytime you gain 10 pounds over your desired weight, immediately lose it.

This is a life-style you can live with and live well.

Chapter Eleven

CHART YOUR SUCCESS!

Each of the preceding chapters instructed you on the how's and why's of developing a comprehensive personal program for maximum, lasting fat loss. But, as was mentioned earlier, it is often difficult to tell if you are making progress! You can potentially be your own worst critic. In order to be sure that you are making progress, you need a system that provides you with objective measures of results. Since it is fat loss that we are after, you require a method of monitoring fat loss. The simplest and most reliable method is the use of skinfold calipers.

Following is a chart of body fat percentages based on gender with aged based ratings.

Age (yrs)					
Rating	20-29	30-39	40-49	50-59	60+
Men*					
Excellent	<11	<12	<14	<15	<16
Good	11-13	12-14	14-16	15-17	16-18
Average	14-20	15-21	17-23	18-24	19-25
Fair	21-23	22-24	24-26	25-27	26-28
Poor	>23	>24	>26	>27	>28
Women**					
Excellent	<16	<17	<18	<19	<20
Good	16-19	17-20	18-21	19-22	20-23
Average	20-28	21-29	22-30	23-31	24-32
Fair	29-31	30-32	31-33	32-34	33-35
Poor	>31	>32	>33	>34	>35

Figure . Chart on Standard Values for Percent Body Fat

(*from Jackson AS, Pollock ML: Generalized equations for predicting body density of men. Br J Nutr, 40:497-504, 1978.)

(**from Jackson AS, Pollock ML, and Ward A: Generalized equations for predicting body density of women. Med Sci Sports Exerc, 12:175-182, 1980.)

Of course, you can monitor your progress by getting your body fat measured by a professional before you begin, and at regular intervals thereafter. However, you need not go to a professional and spend money to attain these measurements. The purpose of this book is to give you all of the tools you need to do everything possible for yourself!

Get a sheet of paper and a writing utensil. You can use the following chart as a template (make copies for future use). Note which side of the body you decide to take measurements from. Some of the measurements are easily made on oneself; others require the aid of a helper. For the sake of consistency and reliability, if possible use the same helper for all future measurements.

Date:_____Time:_____

Weight:_____

Caliper Measurements (mm):

Location	Trial 1	Trial 2	Trial 3	Average
Biceps				
Triceps				
Chest				
Suprailiac				
Subscapular				
2 cm from umbilicus				
Thigh				

To take the skin fold measurement, pinch skin and fat (don't grab the underlying muscle) with your index finger and thumb at the proper location (see description and pictures below). Use your calipers to measure the thickness of the pinched area adjacent to your fingertips. Repeat the measurement three times for each location, and use the average of the three for calculations.

Provided here is a chart for both men and women using the sum of four measurements: the biceps, the triceps, the subscapular and the suprailiac.

Anatomic sites for body fat measurement

Chest	diagonal fold taken one half the distance between the anterior axillary line and the nipple in men or one third the distance from the anterior axillary line in women.
Abdomen	vertical fold taken at a lateral distance of 2 cm from the belly button.
Suprailiac	diagonal fold above the iliac crest where an imaginary line dropped down from the anterior axillary line would meet.
Subscapular	fold taken on diagonal line coming from the vertebral border to 1-2 cm from the inferior angle of the shoulder blade.
Triceps	vertical fold on posterior midline of the upper arm halfway between the acromion process and the elbow.
Thigh	vertical fold on the anterior aspect of the thigh, midway between the hip and knee joints.
Biceps	vertical fold on the anterior aspect of the biceps, midway between the coracoid process and the anterior cubital fossa (the bend at the elbow).

The following are charts for body fat equivalences attained from the sum of the biceps, triceps, suprailiac and subscapular measurements.

MEN	Ages			
Skinfolds (mm)	17-29	30-39	40-49	50+
15	4.8	---	---	---
20	8.1	12.2	12.2	12.6
25	10.5	14.2	15.0	15.6
30	12.9	16.2	17.7	18.6
35	14.7	17.7	19.6	20.8
40	16.4	19.2	21.4	22.9
45	17.7	20.4	23.0	24.7
50	19.0	21.5	24.6	26.5
55	20.1	22.5	25.9	27.9
60	21.2	23.5	27.1	29.2
65	22.2	24.3	28.2	30.4
70	23.1	25.1	29.3	31.6
75	24.0	35.9	30.3	32.7
80	24.8	26.6	31.2	33.8
85	25.5	27.2	32.1	34.8
90	26.2	27.8	33.0	35.8
95	26.9	28.4	33.7	36.6
100	27.6	29.0	34.4	37.4
105	28.2	29.6	45.1	38.2
110	28.8	30.1	35.8	39.0
115	29.4	30.6	36.4	39.7
120	30.0	31.1	37.0	40.4
125	30.5	31.5	37.6	41.1
130	31.0	31.9	38.2	41.8
135	31.5	32.3	38.7	42.4
140	32.0	32.7	39.2	43.0
145	32.5	33.1	39.7	43.6
150	32.9	33.5	40.2	44.1
155	33.3	33.9	40.7	44.6
160	33.7	34.3	41.2	45.1
165	34.1	34.6	41.6	45.6
170	34.5	34.8	42.0	46.1

WOMEN	Ages			
Skinfolds (mm)	17-29	30-39	40-49	50+
15	10.5	—-	—-	—-
20	14.1	17.0	19.8	21.4
25	16.8	19.4	22.2	24.0
30	19.5	21.8	24.5	26.6
35	21.5	23.7	26.4	28.5
40	23.4	25.5	28.2	30.3
45	25.0	26.9	29.6	31.9
50	26.5	28.2	31.0	33.4
55	27.8	29.4	32.1	34.6
60	29.1	30.6	33.2	35.7
65	30.2	31.6	34.1	36.7
70	31.2	32.5	35.0	37.7
75	32.2	33.4	35.9	38.7
80	33.1	34.3	36.7	39.6
85	34.0	35.1	37.5	40.4
90	34.8	35.8	38.3	41.2
95	35.6	36.5	39.0	41.9
100	36.4	37.2	39.7	42.6
105	37.1	37.9	40.4	43.3
110	37.8	38.6	41.0	43.9
115	38.4	39.1	41.5	44.5
120	39.0	39.6	42.0	45.1
125	39.6	40.1	42.5	45.7
130	40.2	40.6	43.0	46.2
135	40.8	41.1	43.5	46.7
140	41.3	41.6	44.0	47.2
145	41.8	42.1	44.5	47.7
150	42.3	42..6	45.0	48.2
155	42.8	43.1	45.4	48.7
160	43.3	43.6	45.8	49.2
165	43.7	44.0	46.2	49.6
170	44.1	44.4	46.6	50.0
175	—-	44.8	47.0	50.4
180	—-	45.2	47.4	50.8

Adapted from: Durnin JVGA and Womersly J, Body fat assessed from total body density and its estimation from skinfold thickness: Measurements on 481 men and women aged 16 to 72 years. Br. J. Nutr., 32:77-97, 1974.

Another method requires only two skin fold measurements. The algorithms are as follows:

For Men:
Body Density = 1.1043 - (0.00133 x thigh skinfold) - (0.00131 x subscapular skinfold)

For Women:
Body Density = 1.0764 - (0.00081 x suprailiac skinfold) - (0.00088 x triceps skinfold)

Fat Percentage = 4.570/Body Density - 4.142 x 100.00

If you do not have access to skinfold calipers, you can use a tape measure to aid in charting your progress. Fill in the chart below, and update the chart on a monthly basis.

Bodypart	Measurement (cm)
Stomach (at belly button)	
Hips	
Arm (largest part)	
Thigh (largest part)	
Neck	

If you have access to a calculator that can calculate logarithms (log) you can use the following formula to get an estimation of your percent bodyfat (Adapated from Hodgdon, J. and Beckett, M. Prediction of percent body fat for U.S. Navy men and women from body circumferences and height. Reports No. 84-29 and 84-11. Naval Health Research Center, San Diego, Cal. 1984.):

WOMEN: %Fat=495/(1.29579-0.35004{log[ABD1+HIP-NECK]})+0.22100(log{HEIGHT})-450

MEN: %Fat=495/(1.0324-0.19077{log[ABD2-NECK]})+0.15456(log{HEIGHT})-450

Where the circumferences (to the nearest .5cm) are:

ABD1: Horizontal, at the level of minimal abdominal width

ABD2: Horizontal at the level of the belly button

HIP: Largest horizontal circumference around the hips

NECK: Inferior to the voice box with the tape sloping slightly downward to the front

HEIGHT: Measured to the nearest .5cm without shoes

As you perform weight lifting, aerobic exercise, and change your eating habits you will be gaining muscle and losing fat. Therefore, your measurements will be just as important to charting your progress as the scale.

Overall, regardless of the method you choose to chart your progress, remember one thing—the number(s) you begin with mean nothing in and of themselves. The real value is in the difference, or change, that occurs from one measurement to the next. Do not let ego get in the way of progress. If you check your numbers and see little to no change, it doesn't signify failure. Utilize the information as feedback to guide your inevitable future success! A lack of progress simply means that you need to modify or alter one or more component of the program. I recommend that you choose one aspect at a time, so that you know which variables affect what result. Sometimes, in order to realize progress, you need only change one small variable, such as increasing your target heart rate by 5% during your aerobic exercise sessions. Be patient and methodical while developing your program. The results will be individualized to you and your body. The information you gather will be well worth the patience and effort!

The following questionnaire may help you assess your health risks. The Body Mass Index (BMI) Chart replaces the old height and weight insurance chart. If you are in the 26-30 category, you are considered overweight. Thirty-one & over is considered obese and a high health risk. The 35 and up category is considered a very high health risk. This does not take into consideration heavily muscled athletic type builds. This group is better assessed through fat percentage.

Weight Wellness Profile

If you are overweight or obese, you have a greater chance of developing serious medical conditions or early death. If you have an established or borderline medical condition, being overweight or obese could worsen that condition. Knowing your weight wellness profile can help you take action to modify your weight properly and improve your health. This profile is designed to encourage discussion with a medical professional. Only your doctor can evaluate the health risks specific to your weight, and recommend appropriate weight management and prevention strategies.

YOUR WEIGHT

1._____ **Body Mass Index (BMI)**
(use BMI calculator or chart following)

less than 25	0 pts.
25 - 29.9	2 pts.
30 - 34.9	3 pts.
35 - 39.9	4 pts.
40 or more	5 pts.

2._____ **Waist Measurement**
(area above hip bone and below rib cage)

Men: less than 40 inches	0 pts.
40 inches or more	2 pts.
Women: less than 35 inches	0 pts.
35 inches or more	2 pts.

YOUR LIFE-STYLE

3._____ **Exercise**
(moderate intensity—such as a brisk walk)

150 minutes or more/week	0 pts.
100 - 149 minutes/week	1 pt.
45 - 99 minutes/week	2 pts.
less than 45 minutes/week	3 pts.

4._____ **Diet**
(I eat fruit, vegetables and low fat foods)

Most of the time	0 pts.
Some of the time	1 pt.
Hardly ever	2 pts.

5._____ **Smoking**

Never smoked	0 pts.
Smoked in the past	1 pt.
Am a smoker now	4 pts.

YOUR MEDICAL HISTORY

6._____ **Diabetes**
(based on fasting blood sugar)

No (less than 110 mg/dl)	0 pts.
Borderline (110-125 mg/dl)	2 pts.
Yes (more than 125 mg/dl)	4 pts.

7._____ **Heart Disease**
(heart attack, bypass surgery, diagnosed angina, or angioplasty—balloon treatment of blocked artery)

No	0 pts.
Yes	5 pts.

8._____ **Blood Pressure**

Normal (less than 130/85)	0 pts.
High Normal (130-139/85-89)	1 pts.
High (140/90 or higher)	3 pts.

9._____ **Cholesterol**

Normal (less than 200 mg/dl)	0 pts.
Borderline (200-239 mg/dl)	1 pt.
High (240 mg/dl or higher)	2 pts.

_____ **TOTAL POINTS**

0 - 3 Points = Keep up the good work! Continue healthy life-style habits to increase your chances of maintaining a healthy weight and preventing several medical conditions.

4 - 9 Points = Preventing weight gain is especially important if you have a medical condition. Visit your doctor regularly for check-ups and maintain a healthy life-style.

10+ Points = Show this profile to your doctor or medical professional and ask about an appropriate plan to manage your weight and medical conditons.

BMI CALCULATOR

Weight (pounds _____ ÷ height^2 (inches x inches) _____

x 704.5 = _____ **your BMI**

BMI CHART Overweight						Obese	
BMI: 25	26	27	28	29	30	35	40
Height (inches)		*Body Weight (pounds)*					
4'10" (58) 119	124	129	134	138	143	167	191
4'11" (59) 124	128	133	138	143	148	173	198
5'0" (60) 128	133	138	143	148	153	179	204
5'1" (61) 132	137	143	148	153	158	185	211
5'2" (62) 136	142	147	153	158	164	191	218
5'3" (63) 141	146	152	158	163	169	197	225
5'4" (64) 145	151	157	163	169	174	204	232
5'5" (65) 150	156	162	168	174	180	210	240
5'6" (66) 155	161	167	173	179	186	216	247
5'7" (67) 159	166	172	178	185	191	223	255
5'8" (68) 164	171	177	184	190	197	230	262
5'8" (69) 169	176	182	189	196	203	236	270
5'10" (70) 174	181	188	195	202	207	243	278
5'11" (71) 179	186	193	200	208	215	250	286
6'0" (72) 184	191	199	206	213	221	258	294
6'1" (73) 189	197	204	212	219	227	265	302
6'2" (74) 194	202	210	218	225	233	272	311
6'3" (75) 200	208	216	224	232	240	279	319
6'4" (76) 205	213	221	230	238	246	287	328

To use this chart: Find your height in the left column. Move across that row toward the right to find your appropriate weight. Then follow eight column up to find your BMI in the black bar at the top.

Chapter Twelve

NUTRITIONAL CHART

FOOD	Wt/Measure	Water	Food Energy	Protein	Fat	Carbohydrate	Calcium	Iron	Vitamin A Value	Thiamin
		Percent	Calories	Grams	Grams	Grams	Milligrams	Milligrams	International Units	Milligrams
DAIRY PRODUCTS										
CHEESE										
Natural Plain	1 oz.	42	100	6	8	1	150	0.1	200	.01
Cheddar, cut pieces	1 oz.	378	115	7	9	Trace	204	2	300	.01
Shredded	1 cup	37	455	28	37	1	815	8	1,200	.03
Cottage Cheese										
Large curd	1 cup	79	235	28	10	6	135	3	370	.05
Small curd	1 cup	79	220	26	9	6	126	3	340	.04
Low fat (2%)	1 cup	79	205	31	4	8	155	4	160	.05
Cream Cheese	1 oz.	54	100	2	10	1	23	.3	400	Trace
Mozzarella	1 oz.	48	90	6	7	1	163	.1	260	Trace
Parmesan, grated	1 cup	18	455	42	30	4	1.37	1.0	700	.05
Provolone	1 tbsp.	18	25	2	2	Trace	69	Trace	40	.02
	1 oz.	41	100	7	8	1	214	.1	230	.01
Ricotta	1 cup	72	430	28	32	7	509	9	1.21	.03
Romano	1 oz.	31	110	9	8	1	302	–	160	–
Swiss	1 oz.	37	105	8	8	1	272	Trace	240	.01
Pasteurized process cheese										
American	1 oz.	39	105	6	9	Trace	174	.1	340	.01
Swiss	1 oz.	42	95	7	7	1	219	.2	230	Trace
CREAM										
Half and half	1 cup	81	315	7	28	10	254	.2	260	.08
	1 tbsp.	81	20	Trace	2	1	16	Trace	20	.01
Whipped topping (preserved)	1 cup	61	155	2	13	7	61	Trace	550	.02
	1 tbsp.	61	10	Trace	1	Trace	3	Trace	30	Trace
Sour Cream	1 cup	71	495	7	48	10	268	1	1.82	.08
	1 tbsp.	71	25	Trace	3	1	14	Trace	90	Trace

FOOD	Wt/Measure	Water	Food Energy	Protein	Fat	Carbohydrate	Calcium	Iron	Vitamin A Value	Thiamin
		Percent	Calories	Grams	Grams	Grams	Milligrams	Milligrams	International Units	Milligrams
Cream continued										
Creamers										
Imitation Powdered	1 tsp.	2	10	Trace	1	1	Trace	Trace	Trace	0
Liquid	1 tbsp.	77	20	Trace	1	2	Trace	10	0	0
MILK										
Whole	1 cup	88	150	8	8	11	291	.1	310	.09
Lowfat (2%)										
No milk solids	1 cup	89	120	8	5	12	297	.1	500	.10
Milk solids added	1 cup	89	125	9	5	12	313	.1	500	.10
Nonfat (skim)										
No milk solids	1 cup	91	85	8	Trace	12	302	.1	500	.09
Milk solids added	1 cup	90	90	9	1	12	316	.1	500	.10
Buttermilk	1 cup	90	100	8	2	12	285	.1	80	.06
Canned Evaporated	1 cup	74	340	17	19	25	657	.5	610	.12
Sweetened Condensed	1 cup	27	980	24	27	166	868	.6	1,000	.28
Dried Buttermilk	1 cup	3	465	41	7	59	1,142	.4	260	.47
Nonfat instant	1 envelope	4	325	32	1	47	1,120	.3	2,160	.38
Chocolate Milk, regular	1 cup	82	210	8	8	26	280	.6	300	.09
Lowfat (2%)	1 cup	84	180	8	5	26	284	.6	500	.10
Eggnog, commercial	1 cup	74	340	10	19	34	330	.5	890	.09
Shakes, Chocolate	1 container	72	355	9	8	63	396	.9	260	.14
Vanilla	1 container	74	350	12	9	56	457	.3	360	.09
Ice Cream	1 cup	61	270	5	14	32	176	.1	540	.05
Frozen Custard	1 cup	60	375	7	23	38	236	.4	790	.08
Ice Milk	1 cup	69	185	5	6	29	176	.1	210	.08
Sherbet	1 cup	66	270	2	4	59	103	.3	190	.03

FOOD	Wt/Measure	Water	Food Energy	Protein	Fat	Carbohydrate	Calcium	Iron	Vitamin A Value	Thiamin
		Percent	Calories	Grams	Grams	Grams	Milligrams	Milligrams	International Units	Milligrams
PUDDING										
Home Recipe Chocolate	1 cup	66	385	8	12	67	250	1.3	390	.05
Vanilla	1 cup	66	285	9	10	41	298	Trace	410	.08
Baked Custard	1 cup	77	305	14	15	29	297	1.1	930	.11
Tapioca Cream	1 cup	72	220	8	8	28	173	.7	480	.07
From Mix—Instant	1 cup	69	235	8	7	63	374	1.3	340	.08
Yogurt with milk solids-fruit	8 oz.	75	230	10	3	42	343	.2	120	.08
Plain	8 oz.	85	145	12	4	16	415	.2	150	.10
With nonfat milk	8 oz.	85	125	13	Trace	17	452	.2	20	.11
EGGS										
Whole large	1	75	80	6	6	1	28	1.0	280	.04
Egg White	1	88	15	3	Trace	Trace	4	Trace	0	Trace
Yolk	1	49	65	3	6	Trace	26	.9	310	.04
Fried in butter	1	72	85	5	6	1	26	.9	290	.03
Hard cooked	1	75	80	6	6	1	26	1.0	260	.04
Poached	1	74	80	6	6	1	28	1.0	260	.04
Scrambled	1	76	95	6	7	1	47	.9	310	.04
FATS & OILS										
Butter	1 stick	16	815	1	92	Trace	27	.2	3,470	.01
	1 tbsp.	16	100	Trace	12	Trace	3	Trace	430	Trace
Whipped	1 stick	16	540	1	61	Trace	18	.1	2,310	Trace
	1 tbsp.	16	65	Trace	8	Trace	2	Trace	290	Trace
Vegetable shortenings	1 tbsp.	0	110	0	13	0	0	0	—	0
Margarine	1 stick	16	815	1	92	Trace	27	.2	3,750	.01
	1 tbsp.	16	100	Trace	12	Trace	3	Trace	470	Trace
Whipped	1 stick	16	545	Trace	61	Trace	18	.1	2,500	Trace
	1 tbsp.	16	70	Trace	8	Trace	2	Trace	310	Trace

FOOD	Wt/Measure	Water (Percent)	Food Energy (Calories)	Protein (Grams)	Fat (Grams)	Carbohydrate (Grams)	Calcium (Milligrams)	Iron (Milligrams)	Vitamin A Value (International Units)	Thiamin (Milligrams)
Fats & Oils continued										
Corn Oil	1 tbsp.	0	120	0	14	0	0	0	—	0
Olive	1 tbsp.	0	120	0	14	0	0	0	—	0
Peanut	1 tbsp.	0	120	0	14	0	0	0	—	0
Soybean, Cottonseed	1 tbsp.	0	120	0	14	0	0	0	—	0
GRAIN PRODUCTS										
Bagel (egg)	1	32	165	6	2	28	9	1.2	30	.14
Biscuit										
Home recipe	1	27	105	2	5	13	34	.4	Trace	.08
From mix	1	29	90	2	3	15	19	.6	Trace	.09
Breadcrumbs—Dry grated	1 cup	7	390	13	5	73	12	3.6	Trace	.35
Breads										
Boston brown	1 slice	45	95	2	1	21	41	.9	—	.06
Cracked wheat	1 slice	35	65	2	1	13	22	.5	Trace	.08
French	1 slice	31	100	3	1	19	15	.8	Trace	.14
Vienna	1 slice	31	75	2	1	14	11	.6	Trace	.10
Italian	1 slice	32	85	3	Trace	17	5	.7	—	.12
Raisin bread	1 slice	35	65	2	1	13	18	.6	Trace	.09
Rye bread										
American light	1 slice	36	60	2	Trace	13	19	.5	—	.07
Pumpernickel	1 slice	34	80	3	Trace	17	27	.8	—	.09
White bread	1 slice	36	70	2	1	13	21	.6	Trace	.10
Whole wheat	1 slice	36	65	3	1	14	24	.8	Trace	.10
BREAKFAST CEREALS										
Hot type, cooked										
Grits, enriched	1 cup	87	125	3	Trace	27	2	.7	Trace	.10
Unenriched	1 cup	87	125	3	Trace	27	2	.2	Trace	.05

FOOD	Wt/Measure	Water	Food Energy	Protein	Fat	Carbohydrate	Calcium	Iron	Vitamin A Value	Thiamin
		Percent	Calories	Grams	Grams	Grams	Milligrams	Milligrams	International Units	Milligrams
Breakfast Cereals continued										
Oatmeal	1 cup	87	130	5	2	23	22	1.4	—	.19
Wheat rolled	1 cup	80	180	5	1	41	19	1.7	—	.17
Ready to eat										
Bran flakes	1 cup	3	105	4	1	28	19	5.6	1,540	.48
Bran flakes with raisins	1 cup	7	145	4	1	40	28	7.9	2,200	—
Corn flakes	1 cup	4	95	2	Trace	21	—	—	—	—
Corn flakes—sugar coated	1 cup	2	155	2	Trace	37	1	—	1,760	.53
Corn—puffed	1 cup	4	80	2	1	16	4	5.7	880	.26
Corn—shredded	1 cup	3	95	2	Trace	22	1	.6	—	.33
Oats—puffed	1 cup	4	60	1	Trace3	13	3	.3	—	.07
Rice—puffed	1 cup	4	60	1	Trace	13	3	.3	—	.07
Wheat flakes	1 cup	4	105	3	Trace	24	12	4.8	1,320	.40
Wheat—puffed	1 cup	3	55	2	Trace	12	4	.6	—	.08
Wheat germ	1 tbsp.	4	25	2	1	3	3	.5	10	.11
CAKES										
Cake mixes with enriched flour										
Angelfood	1 piece	34	135	3	Trace	32	50	.2	—	.03
Coffeecake	1 piece	30	230	5	7	38	44	1.2	120	.14
Cupcakes										
without icing	1	26	90	1	3	14	40	3	40	.05
with icing	1	22	130	2	5	21	47	.4	60	.05
Devil's food with icing	1 piece	24	235	3	8	40	41	1.0	100	.07
Gingerbread	1 piece	37	175	2	4	32	57	.9	Trace	.09
White 2 layer with icing	1 piece	21	250	3	8	45	70	.7	40	.09
Yellow 2 layer with icing	1 piece	26	235	3	8	40	63	.8	100	.06

FOOD	Wt/Measure	Water	Food Energy	Protein	Fat	Carbohydrate	Calcium	Iron	Vitamin A Value	Thiamin
		Percent	Calories	Grams	Grams	Grams	Milligrams	Milligrams	International Units	Milligrams
Cakes continued										
Made from home recipes										
Boston Cream pie										
with custard filling	1 piece	35	210	3	6	34	46	.7	140	.09
Fruit Cake (dark)	1 slice	18	55	1	2	9	11	.4	20	.02
Plain sheet cake without icing	1 piece	25	315	4	12	48	55	.9	150	.13
with icing	1 piece	21	445	4	14	77	61	.8	240	.14
Pound cake	1 piece	16	160	2	10	16	6	.5	80	.05
Sponge cake	1 piece	32	195	5	4	36	20	1.1	300	.09
Brownie—Home recipe	1 brownie	10	95	1	6	10	8	.4	40	.04
From mix	1 brownie	11	85	1	4	13	9	.4	20	.03
Frozen with icing	1 brownie	13	105	1	5	15	10	.4	50	.03
COOKIES										
Chocolate chip from mix	4 cookies	3	200	2	9	29	16	1.0	50	.10
Home recipe	4 cookies	3	105	2	12	24	14	.8	40	.06
Fig bars	4 bars	14	200	2	3	42	44	1.0	60	.04
Gingersnaps	4 cookies	3	90	2	2	22	20	.7	20	.06
Macaroons	2 cookies	4	180	2	9	25	10	.3	—	.02
Oatmeal with raisins	4 cookies	3	235	3	8	38	11	1.4	30	.15
Plain from mix	4 cookies	5	240	2	12	31	17	0.6	30	.10
Sandwich type chocolate										
or vanilla	4 cookies	2	200	2	9	28	10	.7	—	.06
Vanilla wafer	10 cookies	3	185	2	6	30	16	.6	50	.10
CRACKERS										
Graham	2 crackers	6	55	1	1	10	6	.5	—	.02
Rye wafers	2 wafers	6	45	2	Trace	10	7	.5	—	.04
Saltines	4 crackers	4	50	1	1	8	23	.5	—	.05

FOOD	Wt/Measure	Water	Food Energy	Protein	Fat	Carbohydrate	Calcium	Iron	Vitamin A Value	Thiamin
		Percent	Calories	Grams	Grams	Grams	Milligrams	Milligrams	International Units	Milligrams
DANISH										
Pastry	1 pastry	22	275	5	15	30	33	1.2	200	.18
Doughnut, cake type	1 doughnut	24	100	1	5	13	10	.4	20	.05
Glazed	1 doughnut	26	205	3	11	22	16	.6	25	.10
Muffin—Home recipe	1 muffin	39	110	3	4	17	34	.6	90	.09
Bran	1 muffin	35	105	3	4	17	57	1.5	90	.07
Corn	1 muffin	33	125	3	4	19	42	.7	120	.10
Plain	1 muffin	38	120	3	4	17	42	.6	40	.09
PIES										
Apple	1 slice	48	345	3	15	51	11	.9	40	.15
Banana Cream	1 slice	54	285	6	12	40	86	1.0	330	.11
Blueberry	1 slice	51	325	3	15	47	15	1.4	40	.15
Cherry	1 slice	47	350	4	15	52	19	.9	590	.16
Custard	1 slice	58	285	8	14	30	125	1.2	300	.11
Lemon meringue	1 slice	47	305	4	12	45	17	1.0	200	.09
Mince	1 slice	43	365	3	16	56	38	1.9	Trace	.14
Peach	1 slice	48	345	3	14	52	14	1.2	990	.15
Pecan	1 slice	20	495	6	27	61	55	3.7	190	.26
Pumpkin	1 slice	59	275	5	15	32	66	1.0	3,210	.11
Pie crust, home recipe	1 pie shell	15	900	11	60	79	25	3.1	—	.47
ROLLS										
Commercial Brown & Serve	1 roll	27	85	2	2	14	20	.5	Trace	.10
Clover	1 roll	31	85	2	2	15	21	.5	Trace	.11
Hamburger & Frankfurter	1 roll	31	120	3	2	21	30	.8	Trace	.16
Hogie & Submarine	1 roll	31	390	12	4	75	58	3.0	Trace	.54
Home recipe—Clover	1 roll	26	120	3	3	20	16	.7	30	.12

FOOD	Wt/Measure	Water	Food Energy	Protein	Fat	Carbohydrate	Calcium	Iron	Vitamin A Value	Thiamin
		Percent	Calories	Grams	Grams	Grams	Milligrams	Milligrams	International Units	Milligrams
DRY NUTS, SEEDS, RELATED PRODUCTS										
Almonds, chopped	1 cup	5	775	24	70	25	304	6.1	—	.31
Slivered	1 cup	5	690	21	62	22	269	5.4	—	.28
Dry Beans, Navy	1 cup	69	225	15	1	40	95	5.1	—	.27
Red Kidney	1 cup	76	230	15	1	42	74	4.6	10	.13
Lima beans	1 cup	64	260	16	1	49	55	5.9	—	.25
Blackeye peas	1 cup	80	190	13	1	35	43	3.3	30	.40
Brazil nuts	1 oz.	5	185	4	19	3	53	1.0	Trace	.27
Cashew nuts	1 cup	5	785	24	64	41	53	5.3	140	.60
Coconut, fresh shredded	1 cup	51	275	3	28	8	10	1.4	—	.04
Peanuts Roasted in oil	1 cup	2	840	37	72	27	107	3.0	—	.46
Peanut butter	1 tbsp.	2	95	4	8	9	.3	—	.02	.02
Sunflower seeds	1 cup	5	810	35	69	29	174	10.3	70	2.84
Black Walnuts, chopped	1 cup	3	785	26	74	19	Trace	7.5	380	.14
FRUITS & FRUIT PRODUCTS										
Apples, raw	1 apple	84	80	Trace	1	20	10	.4	120	.04
Applesauce, canned sweetened	1 cup	76	230	1	Trace	61	10	1.3	100	.05
unsweetened	1 cup	89	100	Trace	Trace	26	10	1.2	100	.05
Apricots, raw	3 apricots	85	55	1	Trace	14	18	.5	2,890	.03
Canned in syrup	1 cup	77	220	2	Trace	57	28	.8	4,490	.05
Dried	1 cup	25	340	7	1	86	87	7.2	14,170	.01
Avocado, raw	1 avocado	74	370	5	37	13	22	1.3	630	.24
Banana	1	76	100	1	Trace	26	10	.8	230	.06
Banana flakes	1 tbsp.	3	20	Trace	Treace	5	2	.2	50	.01
Blackberries	1 cup	85	85	2	1	19	46	1.3	290	.04
Blueberries	1 cup	83	90	1	1	22	22	1.5	150	.04

Fruit & Fruit Products continued

FOOD	Wt/Measure	Water Percent	Food Energy Calories	Protein Grams	Fat Grams	Carbohydrate Grams	Calcium Milligrams	Iron Milligrams	Vitamin A Value International Units	Thiamin Milligrams
Cherries, sour canned	1 cup	88	105	2	Trace	26	37	.7	1,660	.07
sweet raw	10 cherries	80	45	1	Trace	12	15	.3	70	.03
Cranberry juice	1 cup	83	165	Trace	Trace	42	13	.8	Trace	.03
Cranberry sauce, Sweetened canned	1 cup	62	405	Trace	1	104	17	.6	60	.03
Dates, whole	10 dates	23	220	2	Trace	58	47	2.4	40	.07
Chopped	1 cup	23	490	4	1	130	105	5.3	90	.18
Fruit cocktail, canned in syrup	1 cup	80	195	1	Trace	50	23	1.0	360	.05
Grapefruit, pink or red	1/2	89	50	1	Trace	13	20	5	540	.05
Grapefruit juice—raw, red or white	1 cup	90	95	1	Trace	23	22	.5	—	.10
Frozen concentrate	1 cup	89	100	1	Trace	24	25	.2	20	.10
Grapejuice, canned or bottled	1 cup	83	165	1	Trace	42	28	.8	—	.10
Frozen concentrate	1 cup	86	135	1	Trace	33	8	.3	10	.05
Lemon, raw	1	90	20	1	Trace	6	19	4	10	.03
Lemon juice, raw	1 cup	91	60	1	Trace	20	17	5	50	.07
Frozen from concentrate	1 cup	89	100	Trace	Trace	27	3	Trace	Trace	.11
Cantaloupe	1/2	91	80	2	Trace	20	38	1.1	9,240	.11
Honeydew	1/10	91	50	1	Trace	11	21	.6	60	.06
Orange, whole	1	86	65	1	Trace	16	54	.5	260	.13
Orange juice, raw	1 cup	87	120	2	Trace	26	27	.5	500	.22
Frozen concentrate	1 cup	87	120	2	Trace	29	25	.2	540	.23
Papayas, raw	1 cup	89	55	1	Trace	14	28	.4	2,450	.06
Peaches, raw	1 peach	89	40	1	Trace	10	9	.5	1,330	.02
canned in syrup	1 cup	79	200	1	Trace	51	10	.8	1,100	.03
water packed	1 cup	91	75	1	Trace	20	10	.7	1,100	.02
Pears, raw	1 pear	83	100	1	1	25	13	.5	30	.03
canned in syrup	1 cup	80	195	1	1	50	13	.5	10	.03

FOOD	Wt/Measure	Water	Food Energy	Protein	Fat	Carbohydrate	Calcium	Iron	Vitamin A Value	Thiamin
		Percent	Calories	Grams	Grams	Grams	Milligrams	Milligrams	International Units	Milligrams
Fruit & Fruit Products continued										
Pineapple, raw	1 cup	85	80	1	Trace	21	26	.8	110	.14
canned in syrup	1 cup	80	190	1	Trace	49	28	.8	130	.20
Pineapple juice, unsweetened	1 cup	86	140	1	Trace	34	38	.8	130	.13
Plums, raw	1 plum	87	30	Trace	Trace	8	8	.3	160	.02
Prunes, cooked unsweetened	1 cup	66	255	2	1	67	51	3.8	1,590	.07
Raisins	1 cup	18	420	4	Trace	112	90	5.1	30	.16
Raspberries	1 cup	84	70	1	1	17	27	1.1	160	.11
Strawberries, raw	1 cup	90	55	1	1	13	31	1.5	90	.04
Frozen, sweetened	1 cup	71	310	1	1	79	40	2.0	90	.06
Tangerine, raw	1	87	40	1	Trace	10	34	.3	360	.05
Watermelon, raw	1 wedge	93	110	2	1	27	30	2.1	2,510	.13
VEGETABLES & VEGETABLE PRODUCTS										
Asparagus spears										
From raw	4 spears	94	10	1	Trace	2	13	.4	540	.10
From frozen	4 spears	92	15	2	Trace	2	13	.7	470	.10
Green beans										
Snap from raw	1 cup	92	30	2	Trace	7	63	.8	680	.09
From frozen cuts	1 cup	92	35	2	Trace	8	54	.9	780	.09
French style	1 cup	92	35	2	Trace	8	49	1.2	690	.10
Canned, cuts	1 cup	92	30	2	Trace	7	61	1.2	630	.04
Bean sprouts	1 cup	89	35	4	Trace	7	20	1.4	20	.14
Beets, cooked sliced	1 cup	91	55	2	Trace	12	24	.9	30	.05
Blackeyed peas										
From raw	1 cup	72	180	13	1	30	40	3.5	580	.50
From frozen	1 cup	66	220	15	1	40	43	4.8	290	.19

FOOD	Wt/Measure	Water	Food Energy	Protein	Fat	Carbohydrate	Calcium	Iron	Vitamin A Value	Thiamin
		Percent	Calories	Grams	Grams	Grams	Milligrams	Milligrams	International Units	Milligrams
Vegetables & Vegetable Products *continued*										
Broccoli, from raw	1 stalk	91	45	6	1	8	158	1.4	4,500	.36
From frozen	1 stalk	91	10	1	Trace	1	12	.2	570	.02
Brussel sprouts, from raw	1 cup	88	56	7	1	10	50	1.7	810	.12
From frozen	1 cup	89	50	5	Trace	10	33	1.2	880	.16
Cabbage, shredded from raw	1 cup	92	15	1	Trace	4	34	.3	90	.04
Cabbage celery, from raw	1 cup	95	10	1	Trace	2	32	.5	110	.04
Carrots, from raw	1 carrot	88	30	1	Trace	7	27	.5	7,930	.04
Grated	1 cup	88	45	1	Trace	11	41	.8	12,100	.07
Cauliflower, raw	1 cup	91	31	3	Trace	6	29	1.3	70	.13
Cooked	1 cup	93	30	3	Trace	5	26	.9	80	.11
From frozen	1 cup	94	30	3	Trace	6	31	.9	50	.07
Celery, raw	1 stalk	94	5	Trace	Trace	2	16	.1	110	.01
Collards, raw	1 cup	90	65	7	1	10	367	1.5	14,820	.21
Sweet corn, from raw	1 ear	74	70	2	1	16	2	5	310	.09
From frozen	1 ear	73	120	4	1	27	4	1.0	440	.18
Kernels	1 cup	77	130	5	1	31	5	1.3	580	.15
Canned, cream style	1 cup	76	210	5	2	51	8	1.5	840	.06
Whole kernel	1 cup	76	175	5	1	43	6	1.1	740	.06
Cucumber	8 slices	95	5	Trace	Trace	1	7	.3	70	.01
Lettuce, raw										
Butterhead	1 head	95	25	2	Trace	4	57	3.3	1,580	.10
iceberg	1 head	96	70	5	1	16	108	2.7	1,780	.32
Mushrooms, sliced	1 cup	90	20	2	Trace	3	4	6	Trace	.07
Mustard greens	1 cup	93	30	3	1	6	193	2.5	8,120	.11
Okra pods	10 pods	91	30	2	Trace	6	96	.5	520	.14

Vegetables & Vegetable Products continued

FOOD	Wt/Measure	Water	Food Energy	Protein	Fat	Carbohydrate	Calcium	Iron	Vitamin A Value	Thiamin
		Percent	Calories	Grams	Grams	Grams	Milligrams	Milligrams	International Units	Milligrams
Onions, chopped	1 cup	89	65	3	Trace	15	46	.9	Trace	.05
Young green	6 onions	88	15	Trace	Trace	3	12	.2	Trace	.02
Parsley, raw	1 tbsp.	85	Trace	Trace	Trace	Trace	7	.2	300	Trace
Green peas, canned	1 cup	77	150	8	1	29	44	3.2	1,170	.15
Frozen	1 cup	82	110	8	Trace	19	30	3.0	960	.43
Sweet peppers, raw	1 pod	93	15	1	Trace	4	7	.5	310	.06
Potatoes, baked	1 potato	75	145	4	Trace	33	14	1.1	Trace	.15
French fried	10 strips	45	135	2	7	18	8	.7	Trace	.07
From frozen	10 strips	53	110	2	4	17	5	.9	Trace	.07
Hash browns, from frozen	1 cup	56	345	3	18	45	28	1.9	Trace	.11
Potatoes, mashed	1 cup	83	135	4	2	27	50	8	40	.17
Dehydrated flakes	1 cup	79	195	4	7	30	65	.6	270	.06
Potato chips	10 chips	2	115	1	8	10	8	.4	Trace	.04
Potato salad	1 cup	76	250	7	7	41	80	1.5	350	.20
Radishes, raw	4 radishes	95	5	Trace	Trace	1	5	.2	Trace	.01
Sauerkraut, canned	1 cup	93	40	2	Trace	9	85	1.2	120	.07
Spinach, raw chopped	1 cup	91	15	2	Trace	2	51	1.7	4,460	.06
Summer Squash	1 cup	96	30	2	Trace	7	53	820	.11	1.7
Sweet Potato, baked	1 potato	64	160	2	1	37	46	1.0	9,230	.10
Tomato, raw	1 tomato	94	25	1	Trace	6	16	.6	1,110	.07
Canned	1 cup	94	50	2	Trace	10	14	1.2	2,170	.12
Catsup	1 tbsp.	15	69	15	Trace	4	3	.1	210	.01
Tomato juice, canned	1 cup	95	45	2	Trace	10	17	2.2	1,940	.12
Turnips	1 cup	94	35	1	Trace	8	54	.6	Trace	.06
Greens	1 cup	94	30	3	Trace	5	252	1.5	8,270	.15

FOOD	Wt/Measure	Water	Food Energy	Protein	Fat	Carbohydrate	Calcium	Iron	Vitamin A Value	Thiamin
		Percent	Calories	Grams	Grams	Grams	Milligrams	Milligrams	International Units	Milligrams
FISH, MEAT, POULTRY										
Clams, raw	3 oz.	82	65	11	1	2	59	5.2	90	.08
Crabmeat, canned	1 cup	77	135	24	3	1	61	1.1	—	.11
Fish sticks	1 stick	66	50	5	3	2	3	.1	—	.01
Haddock, fried	3 oz.	66	140	17	5	5	34	1.0	—	.03
Ocean Perch	1 fillet	59	195	16	11	6	28	1.1	—	.10
Oysters, raw	1 cup	85	160	20	4	8	226	13.2	740	.34
Salmon, Pink canned	3 oz.	71	120	17	5	—	167	.7	60	.03
Sardines, canned	3 oz.	62	175	20	9	—	372	2.5	190	.02
Shad, baked	3 oz.	64	170	20	10	—	20	.5	30	.11
Shrimp, canned	3 oz.	70	100	21	1	1	98	2.6	50	.01
Tuna, canned	3 oz.	61	170	24	7	—	7	1.6	70	.04
Tuna salad	1 cup	70	350	30	22	7	41	2.7	590	.08
Bacon, fried	2 slices	8	85	4	8	Trace	2	.5	—	.06
Ground beef	3 oz.	60	185	23	10	—	10	3.0	20	.08
Roast, baked	3 oz.	40	375	17	33	—	8	2.2	70	.05
Steak, broiled	3 oz.	44	330	20	27	—	9	2.5	50	.05
Corn beef, canned	3 oz.	59	185	22	10	—	17	3.7	—	.01
Corn beef hash	1 cup	67	400	19	25	24	29	4.4	—	.02
Beef vegetable stew	1 cup	82	220	16	11	15	29	2.9	2,400	.15
Beef potpie	1 piece	55	515	21	30	39	29	3.8	1,720	.30
Chili con carne	1 cup	72	340	19	16	31	82	4.3	150	.06
Lamb chop	3.1 oz.	43	360	18	32	—	8	1.0	—	.11
Roasted leg	3 oz.	54	235	22	16	—	9	1.4	—	.13
Shoulder roast	3 oz.	50	285	18	23	—	9	1.0	—	.11
Cured Ham	3 oz.	54	245	18	19	—	8	2.2	—	.40
Luncheon meat	1 oz.	59	65	5	5	—	3	.8	—	.12

FOOD	Wt/Measure	Water	Food Energy	Protein	Fat	Carbohydrate	Calcium	Iron	Vitamin A Value	Thiamin
		Percent	Calories	Grams	Grams	Grams	Milligrams	Milligrams	International Units	Milligrams
Fish, Meat, Poultry continued										
Canned	1 slice	55	175	9	15	1	5	1.3	—	.10
Pork roast	3 oz.	46	310	21	24	—	9	2.7	—	.78
Pork shoulder	3 oz.	46	320	20	26	—	9	2.6	—	.46
Bologna	1 slice	56	85	3	8	Trace	2	.5	—	.05
Deviled Ham, canned	1 tbsp.	51	45	2	4	—	1	.3	—	.02
Frankfurter	1	57	170	7	15	1	3	.8	—	.08
Salami, cooked	1 slice	51	90	5	7	Trace	3	.7	—	.07
Vienna sausage	1	63	40	2	3	Trace	1	.3	—	.01
Veal cutlet	3 oz.	80	185	23	9	—	9	2.7	—	.06
Chicken breast	2.8 oz.	58	160	26	5	1	9	1.3	70	.04
Drumstick, fried	1.3 oz.	55	90	12	4	Trace	6	.9	50	.03
Chicken a la king	1 cup	68	470	27	34	12	127	2.5	1,130	.10
Chicken & noodles, home recipe	1 cup	71	365	22	18	26	26	2.2	430	.05
Chicken chow mein, canned	1 cup	89	95	7	Trace	18	45	1.3	150	.05
Home recipe	1 cup	78	255	31	10	10	58	2.5	280	.08
Turkey, roasted										
Dark meat	4 slices	61	175	26	7	—	—	2.0	—	.03
Light meat	4 slices	62	150	28	3	—	—	1.0	—	.04
SPAGHETTI										
Served hot	1 cup	73	155	5	1	32	11	1.3	—	.20
In tomato sauce with cheese										
Home recipe	1 cup	77	260	9	9	37	80	2.3	1,080	.25
Canned	1 cup	80	190	6	2	39	40	2.8	930	.35
With meat balls & tomato sauce										
Home recipe	1 cup	70	330	19	12	39	124	3.7	1,590	.25
Canned	1 cup	78	260	12	10	29	53	3.3	1,000	.15

FOOD	Wt/Measure	Water	Food Energy	Protein	Fat	Carbohydrate	Calcium	Iron	Vitamin A Value	Thiamin
		Percent	Calories	Grams	Grams	Grams	Milligrams	Milligrams	International Units	Milligrams
SUGARS & SWEETS										
Caramels	1 oz.	8	115	1	3	22	42	.4	Trace	.01
Milk Chocolate	1 oz.	1	145	2	9	16	65	.3	80	.10
Chocolate Peanuts	1 oz.	1	160	5	12	11	33	.4	Trace	.10
Fudge	1 oz.	8	115	1	3	21	22	.3	Trace	.01
Gum Drops	1 oz.	12	100	Trace	Trace	25	2	.1	—	—
Marshmallows	1 oz.	17	90	1	Trace	23	5	.5	—	—
Honey	1 tbsp.	17	65	Trace	—	17	1	.1	—	Trace
Jams & Preserves	1 tbsp.	29	55	Trace	Trace	14	4	.2	Trace	Trace
Jellies	1 tbsp.	29	50	Trace	Trace	13	4	.3	Trace	Trace
Chocolate Syrup, Fudge type	2 tbsp.	25	125	2	5	20	48	.5	60	.02
Molasses	1 tbsp.	24	45	—	—	11	137	3.2	—	.02
Brown Sugar	1 cup	2	820	—	—	121	187	7.5	—	.02
Granulated White	1 cup	1	270	—	—	199	—	.2	—	—
Powdered	1 cup	1	366	—	—	100	—	.1	—	—
MISCELLANEOUS										
Baking Powder	1 tsp.	2	5	Trace	Trace	1	58	—	—	—
Barbeque Sauce	1 cup	81	230	4	17	20	53	2.0	900	.03
Beer	12 oz.	92	150	1	—	14	18	Trace	—	.01
Gin, Rum, Vodka, Whiskey 90 proof	1.5 oz.	62	110	—	—	Trace	—	—	—	—
Wine, table	3.5 oz.	86	85	Trace	—	4	9	.4	—	Trace
Carbonated Water	12 oz.	92	115	—	—	37	—	—	—	—
Ginger Ale	12 oz.	92	115	—	—	29	—	—	—	—
Gelatin	1 cup	84	140	4	—	34	—	—	—	—
Mustard, prepared	1 tsp.	80	5	Trace	Trace	Trace	4	.1	—	—
Green Olives	4	78	15	Trace	2	Trace	8	.2	40	—

FOOD	Wt/Measure	Water	Food Energy	Protein	Fat	Carbohydrate	Calcium	Iron	Vitamin A Value	Thiamin
		Percent	Calories	Grams	Grams	Grams	Milligrams	Milligrams	International Units	Milligrams
Miscellaneous continued										
Pickles, fresh	2 slices	79	10	Trace	Trace	3	5	.3	20	Trace
Sweet	1 pickle	61	20	Trace	Trace	5	2	.2	10	Trace
Tomato soup	1 cup	84	175	7	7	23	168	.8	1,200	.10
Beef noodle	1 cup	93	65	4	3	7	7	1.0	50	.05
Clam chowder	1 cup	92	80	2	3	12	34	1.0	880	.02
Cream of Mushroom	1 cup	90	135	2	10	10	41	.5	70	.02
Brewer's Yeast	1 tbsp.	5	25	3	Trace	3	17	1.4	Trace	1.25
Salad Dressing										
Blue Cheese	1 tbsp.	32	75	1	8	1	12	Trace	30	Trace
French	1 tbsp.		39	65	Trace	6	3	.2	.1	—
Italian	1 tbsp.	28	85	Trace	9	1	2	Trace	Trace	Trace
Toaster Pastries	1 pastry	12	200	3	6	36	54	1.9	500	.16
Waffle, Home recipe	1 waffle	41	210	7	7	28	85	1.3	250	.17
Mix	1 waffle	42	205	7	8	27	179	1.0	170	.14
Flour, wheat sifted	1 cup	12	420	12	1	88	18	3.3	—	.74
Cake flour	1 cup	12	350	7	1	76	16	2.8	—	.61
Self rising	1 cup	12	440	12	1	93	331	3.6	—	.80
Cornmeal—whole ground	1 cup	12	435	11	5	90	24	2.9	620	.46
Pizza, cheese	1 slice	45	145	6	4	22	86	1.1	230	.16
Popcorn with oil	1 cup	3	40	1	2	5	1	.2	—	—
Sugar coated	1 cup	4	135	2	1	30	2	.5	—	—
Pretzel, Dutch twist	1 pretzel	5	60	2	1	12	4	.2	—	.05
Pretzel, Thin twist	10 pretzels	5	235	6	3	46	13	.9	—	.20
Egg noodles	1 cup	71	200	7	2	37	16	1.4	110	.22
Rice, white instant, Long grain cooked	1 cup	73	225	4	Trace	50	21	1.8	—	.23
Parboiled	1 cup	73	185	4	Trace	41	33	1.4	—	.19

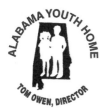

Alabama Youth Home

The Alabama Youth Home Now Cares For Over 100 Boys and Girls Each Year!

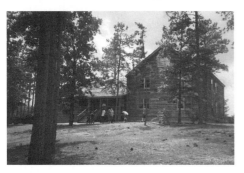

Boys' Home #1 in Westover

The Boys' Group Homes

We have two boys' homes located in the Chelsea/Westover area of Shelby County. The boys' home is a big log cabin with a barn, two lakes, and lots of animals. Keeping the farm atmosphere going requires a lot of daily chores. That, along with a regular exercise program helps teach discipline and responsibility to each boy there.

We also have a boys' group home in Elmore County in the Montgomery area. This boys' home is licensed for 12 boys and also has the same type of discipline and responsibility programs.

All the boys and girls are involved in church and a wholesome Christian atmosphere.

The Girls' Group Home

The Girls' Home is also located in the Chelsea/Westover area. This home provides a resident treatment facility to girls during a particularly difficult time in their lives. The girls are encouraged in a Christian atmosphere through good, sound counseling and academic help. They also have the ability to develop self-confidence and expand their interest through a variety of learning experiences and healthy activities. They are able to live in a family-like atmosphere, while learning self-discipline and handling adversity in life.

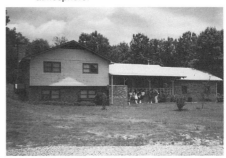

Westover Girls' Home

"Providing kids the help they need through your sponsorship"

Camp Prevention
on Lake Martin

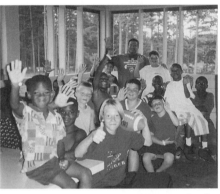

It is time to stop waiting for the problem to occur and then trying to fix it! Wouldn't it be better to **prevent** a child from becoming delinquent rather than waiting until it's too late? The Alabama Youth Home has expanded its ministry. into the area of Juvenile Delinquency and Drop Out Prevention. We have a beautiful 25-acre camp on Lake Martin including a peninsula and recreation area on the water. The camp itself can house

Smiling faces and changed lives—that's what Camp Prevention is all about!

over 50 boys at a time in rustic but adequate facilities. The therapeutic camping environment promotes healthy living in a Christian atmosphere, encouraging the children to stay in school and out of trouble. These children will also receive a personalized monthly newsletter, a Christmas and Birthday gift from The Director, further encouraging them while they are away from camp. We target children that are at risk of becoming delinquent, and feel this will have a major impact on their lives. Prevention is something that Alabama has not focused on and, with your help, these boys will become tomorrow's leaders instead of tomorrow's delinquents.

"An ounce of prevention is worth a pound of cure"

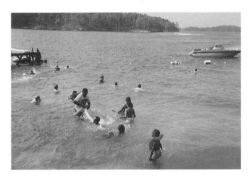

Lake Martin is a beautiful setting for our camp to have a lifelong impact on these boys.

"Taking at-risk children and building tomorrow's leaders"

Our Counselors

Both the boys' and girls' homes have wonderful, Christian staff members who have been together for years. Tom has been privileged to work with many of his staff for over ten years. These dedicated Christian workers have a missionary zeal, compassion, and commitment (working together with your help) to see these young lives changed forever.

Our camp also has wonderful staff members who are dedicated not only to teaching these boys life changing lessons, but showing them how to have good, clean fun. We are very fortunate to have these gifted people on our team!

The Founder & Director

The Alabama Youth Home's founder and director, Dr. Tom Owen, since 1975 has devoted his life to helping troubled and hurting children and bringing their plight to public awareness. Tom has a degree in Health and Juvenile Justice, a Masters and an Ed.S in Counseling Psychology from the University of Alabama at Birmingham. He is a licensed professional counselor and holds a Doctorate in Christian Counseling. Tom does group therapy in the homes each week, concentrating on anger management, self control, and living a healthy, productive Christian life. He also speaks to each group of campers at Camp Prevention.

Tom has been featured many times on national television as a professional strongman, performs all over the world, and is one of the few weight lifters in history to be pictured in the *Guinness Book of World Records*. Also, is a first runner-up in the Mr. America contest. Tom uses his professional strongman feats as a means to raise funds for the Alabama Youth Home and to make the public aware of Alabama's hurting and troubled children.

Thank you for your support! Our boys and girls are supported by your gifts and contributions!

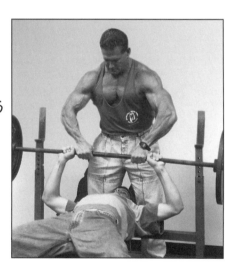

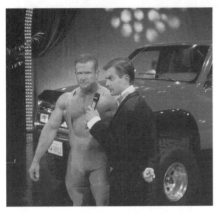

Tom appears on the Comedy Central program *Viva Variety* in August 1998.

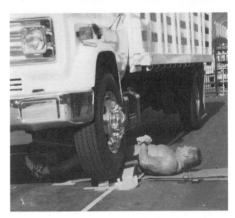

Tom gets run over by a truck on the *Crook & Chase Show* on the CBS Network.

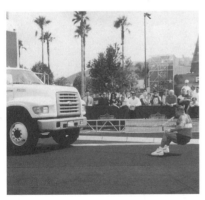

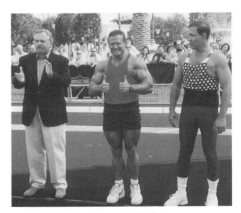

Prior to the Crook & Chase Show, Tom appeared on the Fox Network's *WOW II - World's Most Awesome Acts*, with Cliff from *Cheers* hosting.

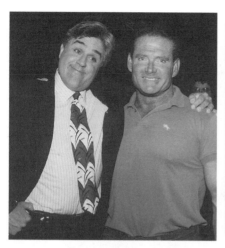

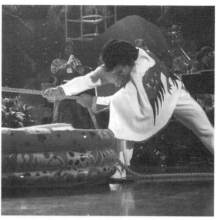

Tom also was featured on The Tonight Show with Jay Leno as a "Big Elvis" who competed against five smaller Elvi in a tug-of-war match. Tom pulled the smaller Elvi into a tub of Elvis' favorite dessert—banana pudding!

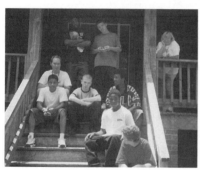

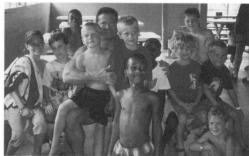

Tom, "Mr. Muscle" as he is known on television, is one of the most sought after professional strongmen, making appearances both here and abroad.
This continues to be an excellent way to bring the plight of hurting children to public awareness and to raise much needed funds for these kids.

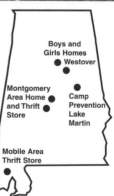

Boys and
Girls Homes
● Westover
●

Montgomery
Area Home ●
and Thrift
Store

Camp
Prevention
Lake
Martin
●

Mobile Area
Thrift Store
●

It's all for the kids!
Thanks for helping!

You Can Help!

The Alabama Youth Home and Camp Prevention are funded through your gifts and contributions. We appreciate vehicles, monetary gifts or any donation to help support these children. **Monthly gifts are extremely helpful to us. We can assist you in making monthly contributions through our bank draft service. Please call us for details!**

This gift of $_____ is made
___in honor of   ___in memory of (please check one)
_____.
Please send an acknowledgment card to:
Name(s)_____
Address_____
My name should appear as_____
Please mail to:
Alabama Youth Home, PO Box 66, Westover, Al 35185

If you would like to give a gift in honor or memory of someone, simply fill out the information above and return. This would be a great gift for any holiday or occasion, such as birthdays or anniversaries. Memorial gifts can be anywhere from a small gift that will get an acknowledgment card to a large gift that would name a building after the person or the donor.

Other ways you can help include remembering the Alabama Youth Home in your will or through insurance bequests. There are also great tax advantages in donating vehicles or appreciated items such as real estate, stocks, or anything else of value, as well as establishing charitable remainder trusts. For more information on these types of donations, please call Dr. Tom Owen at 205-991-9311 or write him at 4500 Valleydale Road, Suite 160, Birmingham, AL 35242.

The Alabama Youth Home is a non-profit 501c(3) corporation and is controlled by a volunteer Board of Directors and gets an opinion audit every year. Our sales tax exemption code is #EX-8698.

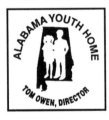

Alabama Youth Home
Westover, AL 35185